BOOST YOUR IMMUNE SYSTEM

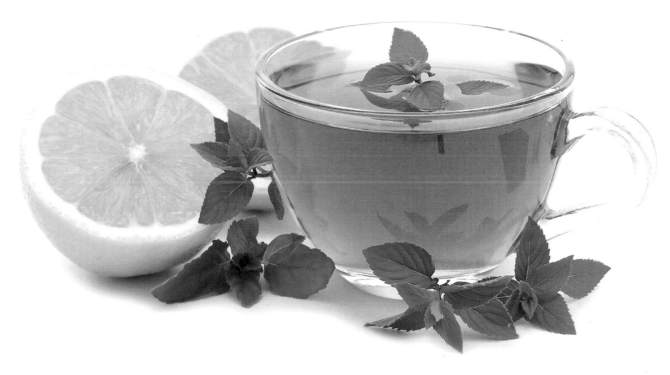

Publications International, Ltd.

TABLE OF CONTENTS

INTRODUCTION

You're feeling run down. Or you've got the sniffles…again…or a lingering cough from your last cold. You've been wondering: how can you avoid colds? How can you boost your health in the long term to prevent inflammation, cancer, and other diseases? How can you reach and stay at your best health, enjoying high energy and avoiding fatigue?

The good news is, you can take steps to do all those things. And some relatively simple steps can pay huge dividends, both immediately and in the long term. In *Boost Your Immune System,* we'll look at the strategies you can take to bolster your immune system and improve your health. Here's just a preview of what's in store:

In chapter 1, "Starting Off," we'll look at the basics of how the immune system works—and what happens when things go wrong. This chapter includes "20 Fast Fixes" to get you started in boosting your immune system.

Chapter 2, "Sleep Well, Live Better," examines the links between good sleep and good health. It turns out that those eight hours a night help you out 24 hours a day! And if you're not getting good sleep, this chapter offers some suggestions for practicing good sleep hygiene to get deep, restorative sleep.

Mental stress has big effects on the body and the immune system. Chapter 3, "Healthy Mind, Healthy Body," explores strategies for stress reduction, including mindfulness, gratitude, meditation, active relaxation techniques, exercise, and more. A positive attitude can have positive effects!

What you take into your body can have a big effect on your immune system and your health. Chapters 4 and 5, "Eating for Better Health," and "Healing Herbs, Vitamins, and Supplements," give tips on boosting your immune system through eating a healthy diet, as well as specific foods, herbs, vitamins, and supplements that can offer health benefits. From general guidelines on nutrition to more specific discussions about chocolate, olive oil, tea, garlic, and ginger, we'll take a closer look at how what you ingest shapes how you feel.

Chapter 6, "An Ounce of Prevention," puts the focus on environmental factors such as air and water quality and preventive medicine such as vaccines. From water filters to the flu shot, we'll look at steps you can take to prevent future health problems.

In the final chapter, "Getting Over It Quickly," we'll give you some strategies for when you do get sick. Learn specific strategies on how to deal with allergies, colds, flu, food poisoning and other gastrointestinal troubles, bronchitis, anemia, and more. Learn how you can ease your symptoms and give your immune system a hand as it fights off infections. Best of all, many of these strategies rely on simple, inexpensive items that you may already have in your kitchen or around the house.

Our health is one of our most precious resources. It only makes good sense to foster good health. And you'll be amazed at how much you can do with simple lifestyle changes!

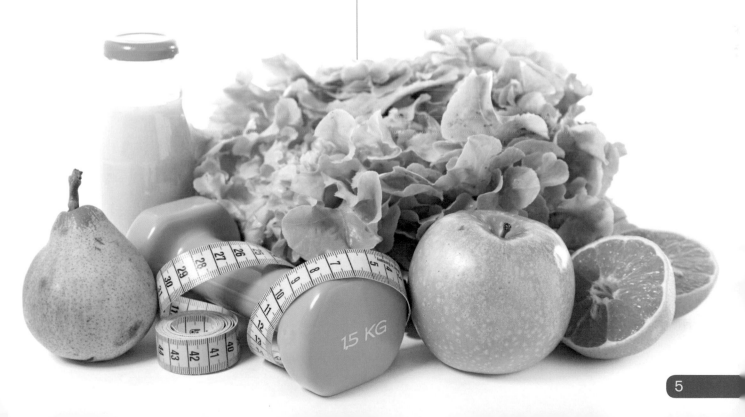

STARTING OFF

WHAT IS IMMUNITY?

In medical terms, having immunity means that you have resistance to infection or a specified disease. If you have low immunity, it means your immune system isn't up to par and that you have a greater chance of getting the germ-du-jour. There are many factors that affect your body's response to a foreign invader, including how you're feeling at the moment you're introduced to a suspect germ. But if you consistently end up with the latest flu bug or stomach virus, your immune system may just be running on empty.

THE BATTLE FOR YOUR BODY

Imagine your immune system as the front line in your body's war against foreign invaders. The vast network of glands, tissues, and cells are all soldiers working together to get rid of bacteria, viruses, parasites, and anything that invades their turf. The major troops in this war are the lymphatic system, made of the lymph nodes, thymus, spleen, and tonsils; white blood cells; and other specialized cells such as macrophages and mast cells. Each of these troops has a specialized job in enhancing the body's ability to fight off infection.

Lymph nodes are responsible for filtering out waste products from tissues throughout the body. Under the lymph nodes' command are cells that overtake bacteria and other potentially harmful foreign bodies and crush them like ants. That's why your lymph nodes swell up like golf balls when you are actively fighting off an infection.

Science has long told moms that breast-feeding their babies could help them avoid infections, but how does breast milk work to boost tiny immune systems? Breast milk actually triggers growth in the thymus gland—a vital component to fending off infection. One study found that babies who were breast-fed had a thymus gland that was twenty times larger than formula-fed babies.

The thymus is your immune system's stealth warfare command center. You may not spend much time thinking of your thymus—you may not even be clear about where it is in your body—but without it you would be one sick puppy. (It's behind your sternum, incidentally, between your lungs.) The thymus is a gland that produces many of those disease-fighting foot soldiers—the white blood cells that come to your defense against many types of infections. And the thymus produces hormones that enhance your immune function overall. So if your thymus isn't working as it should, your body may have trouble fighting off infection successfully.

The spleen, found on the left side of your body near your stomach, is vital to your immune defense. It produces white blood cells, kills bacteria, and enhances the immune system overall. White blood cells are your body's main defense in the battle against infection. White blood cells with names such as neutrophils, eosinophils, basophils, T cells, B cells, and natural killer cells, are all part of the vast army of disease assaulters.

WHEN THE ENEMY STRIKES

When something enters your body that is viewed by the immune system as harmful, your body goes into a state of heightened alert. When your immune system is healthy and all systems are go,

LIVING WITHOUT A SPLEEN

Sometimes, due to physical trauma such as a car accident, or because of certain blood disorders or cancers, the spleen is removed in a procedure called a splenectomy. People can live without a spleen, relying on other organs to take up its work—but it does compromise their immune system. Before a spleen removal, doctors may recommend a set of vaccines in order to stave off anticipated problems.

these foreign invaders, or antigens, are typically met by a barrage of antibodies, which are produced by white blood cells. These antibodies latch on to antigens and set into action all the events that lead to the invader's eventual demise. If things in your immune system are not working properly, you become less able to fight off those foreign invaders. Eventually they set up shop in your body and you get sick. An impaired immune system can make you more susceptible to colds and other merely frustrating illnesses, but it can also make you more at risk for developing cancer.

Ironically, the symptoms that vex us are often signals of our body fighting back. For example, a cough is produced when viruses, bacteria, dust, pollen, or other foreign substances irritate respiratory passages in the throat and lungs. The cough reflex is the body's effort to rid the passageways of such intruders, and it spares no power in the expulsion. A cough reflex can expel a foreign substance at velocities as high as 100 miles per hour. In a similar way, fever is your body's attempt to kill off invading bacteria and other nasty organisms that can't survive the heat. The hypothalamus, which is the body's thermostat, senses the assault on the body and turns up the heat much the way you turn up the thermostat when you feel cold. It's a simple defense mechanism, and the sweat that comes with a fever is merely a way to cool the body down.

It used to be standard medical practice to knock that fever out as quickly as possible. Not so anymore. The value of fever is recognized, and since a fever will usually subside when the infection that's causing it runs its course, modern thinking is to ride out that fever, especially if it stays under 102°F in adults. However, if a fever is making you uncomfortable or interfering with your ability to eat, drink, or sleep, treat it. Your body needs adequate nutrition, hydration, and rest to fight the underlying cause of the fever. For more tips on fighting back against cold and flu, see the final chapter.

INHERITED OR ACQUIRED?

Is immunity inherited or acquired? The answer is...both. There are two basic types of immunity. Natural immunity is the type you inherit from your parents. If your mom and dad rarely miss a day's work and are the picture of health, chances are that you will be, too. But no matter how good your genes are, if you don't exercise or eat right and are chronically stressed, you could increase your chances of getting sick.

The second type of immunity is active immunity. Active immunity means you become immune to a disease because you had it already, like the chicken pox, or because you got a vaccination against the disease, such as your annual flu shot.

ALTERNATIVE TRADITIONS

The idea that health depends on both genetics and lifestyle choices is not limited to Western medicine. In traditional Chinese medicine, qi is an extremely important concept. Although qi plays a central role in traditional Chinese medicine, it is extremely difficult to define. It is best to understand it in terms of its functions and activities, where it is more readily perceived. Situated somewhere between matter and energy, qi has the qualities of both. It has substance without structure, and it possesses energy qualities but can't be measured. It is the fundamental power underlying all the activities of nature as well as the vital life force of the human body. Chinese medicine traditionally divides qi into various types, depending on its source and function. The original source of this life force is a person's parents, and the qi inherited from them is known as prenatal qi. Prenatal qi, the basic constitution of a human being, depends on genetics and the quality of the parents' lives at the time of conception and during pregnancy. This qi initially locates in and around the kidneys. As the organs of the body begin to function autonomously, the prenatal qi moves into the rest of the body. This qi is the person's heritage, and it cannot be replenished; however, healthy lifestyle, diet, and breathing practices can conserve prenatal qi and slow down its depletion. Preservation of prenatal qi is one of the most important contributions of traditional Chinese medicine. It enables a person who is sickly and weak to live a life of health and vitality. The process involves a simultaneous conservation of prenatal qi with practices that enhance the formation of postnatal qi. Postnatal qi, or acquired qi, is derived from the digestion of food and extracted from the air we breathe. Combined with prenatal qi, it forms the totality of the body's power to perform all the vital processes of life.

20 FAST FIXES

You can't change the natural immunity you inherited. But you can build your immune system. In the rest of this chapter, we'll look at 20 quick ways you can improve your immunity. One thing you'll notice is that many are food based. Science is constantly proving that getting enough of the right nutrients can help you preserve your health. Scientific studies are discovering that avoiding something as simple as a cold or something as life threatening as cancer may all be affected by what you stock in your kitchen and put in your stomach.

1. **Almonds.** Eat a handful of almonds for your daily dose of vitamin E. E is an immune-strengthening antioxidant, and studies have found that vitamin E deficiency causes major problems in the integrity of the immune system.

2. **Crab.** A zinc deficiency can zap your immune system. Zinc acts as a catalyst in the immune system's killer response to foreign bodies, and it protects the body from damage from invading cells. It also is a necessary ingredient for white blood cell function. Nosh on 3 ounces fresh or canned crab and you've got one-third of your recommended daily allowance (RDA) of this immune-enhancing nutrient.

3. **Navy beans.** Everybody needs a little folic acid (it's the most common nutrient deficiency in the United States). And not getting enough of this vital nutrient can actually shrink vital immune system fighters like your thymus and lymph nodes. To make sure you're getting your fill of folic acid, try popping open a can of navy beans with dinner. One cup gets you half of your recommended daily allowance (RDA) of folic acid.

4. **Guava.** Go a little tropical with this tasty fruit and get more than twice your daily vitamin C needs. Vitamin C acts as an immune enhancer by helping white blood cells perform at their peak and quickening the response time of the immune system.

5. **Yellow bell pepper.** Bell peppers are another powerhouse source of vi-

tamin C. Bell peppers, especially the yellow ones have more vitamin C than oranges.

6. **Chicken.** Selenium is a trace mineral that is vital to the development and movement of white blood cells in the body. A 3-ounce piece of chicken will give you almost half your daily needs.

7. **Pork.** Not getting enough vitamin B_6 can keep your immune system from functioning at its

best. Eating 3 ounces of lean roast pork will provide you with one-third of most adults' daily requirements for this immune-helping vitamin.

8. **Wine.** Have a glass of red wine and you may help your body take out a few potentially harmful foreign bodies. Certain components in wine seem to be helpful in killing infectious bacteria, such as salmonella. But be careful. Drinking too much alcohol can cause your immune system to become depressed, leaving you more open to infection. A glass a day should do the trick.

LET THEM DRINK WINE

During a cholera epidemic in Paris in the late 19th century, a French doctor discovered that people who drank wine were more immune to the dreaded disease. He asked people to mix wine into their water to protect themselves against the deadly plague.

9. **Yogurt.** We'll explore the benefits of yogurt in more detail in chapters 4 and 7. Yogurt seems to have a marked effect on the immune system. It strengthens white blood cells and helps the immune system produce antibodies. One study found that people

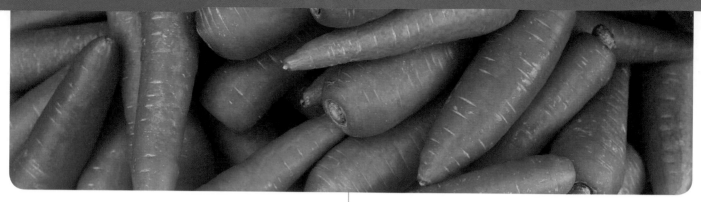

who ate 6 ounces of yogurt a day avoided colds, hay fever, and diarrhea. Another study found that yogurt could be an ally in the body's war against cancer.

10.   Echinacea. Research has shown echinacea to boost the body's immune response. It is particularly effective at fighting viral infections, such as the cold and flu, helping your body heal faster. Take 1 or 2 capsules or tablets up to three times a day. You can also buy dried echinacea and brew it into a tea. Simmer 1 to 2 teaspoons in 1 cup boiling water for 10 to 15 minutes; drink up to 3 cups a day. Find out more in chapter 5.

11.   Carrots. Carotenes, like the beta-carotene found in carrots and other red, yellow, orange, and dark-green leafy vegetables, are the protectors of the immune system, specifically the thymus gland. Carotenes strengthen white blood cell production, and numerous studies have shown that eating foods rich in beta-carotene helps the body fight off infection more easily.

12.   Garlic. Garlic is well-known for its antibacterial and antiviral properties. It's even been thought to help prevent cancer. Researchers think these benefits stem from garlic's amazing effect on the immune system. One study found that people who ate more garlic had more of the natural killer white blood cells than those who did not eat garlic.

13.   Kale. A cup of kale will give you your daily requirement of vitamin A.

Vitamin A is an antioxidant that helps your body fight cancer cells and is essential in the formation of white blood cells. Vitamin A also increases the ability of antibodies to respond to invaders.

14. **Shiitake mushrooms.** Throw a few shiitake mushrooms in your stir-fry and you may prevent your yearly cold. Scientists have discovered that specific components of shiitake mushrooms boost your immune system and act as antiviral agents.

15. **Skip the sugar.** Sugar may keep your white blood cells from being their strongest. Keep the sweet stuff to a minimum if your immune system isn't working like it should.

16. **Forgo fat.** Polyunsaturated fats in vegetable oils such as corn, safflower, and sunflower oil seem to be a deterrent to an efficiently running immune system.

17. **Lose a few pounds.** Being overweight has a major effect on your immune system. One study found that the white blood cells in overweight people weren't as able to fight off infection as those of their healthy-weight peers.

18. **Try to relax.** If stress causes you to lose your cool, you could be impairing your immune system. Chronic stress can even shrink your thymus gland, creating major problems in your body's ability to fight off infection. This is probably why you get a horrible cold after you finish a big project at work. Of course, relaxing is easier said than done, so we'll look at this in more detail in chapter 3.

19. **Add some activity.** Exercise is a proven immune system booster. Don't overdo it, though. Too much can wear you down and create immune system problems.

20. **Get your yearly flu shot.** This applies especially for the young and the elderly, and anyone with a compromised immune system. But since 2010, the CDC has recommended

that, "Everyone 6 months of age and older should get a flu vaccine every season." Not only will can it keep you from a miserable week, but it can keep you from passing it along to someone with a compromised immune system. Many insurance plans now cover this shot.

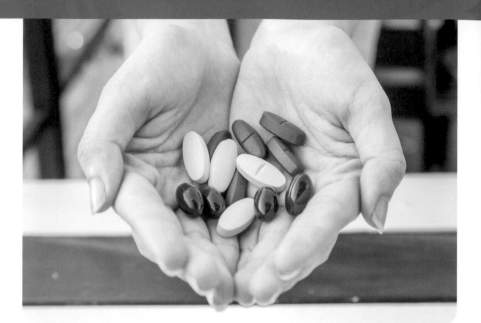

THE ROLE OF MULTIVITAMINS

Getting enough of essential nutrients is a good start on the road to a healthy immune system. And generally, eating a well-balanced diet will get you on that road. But you may be thinking about taking a multivitamin to help fill in the gaps. Are they worth it? And what should you look for? Most nutrition experts would tell you to get the majority of your nutrients from food—mostly because there are other good-for-you components in food that a specific vitamin may not offer. Taking a multivitamin is a good backup plan. If you decide to take a multivitamin, follow these tips:

- Look for a vitamin/mineral combination. You need vitamins and minerals to enhance your immune system, so be sure the product you choose has all you need.

- Don't use products that have more than 100 percent of the recommended daily allowance (RDA) or daily value (DV) of a nutrient. You're going to get most of your vitamins and minerals from your diet, so don't go overboard.

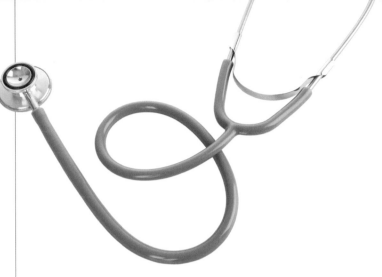

- Make sure your multivitamin meets your needs. If you need to boost your immune system, look for a multivitamin that has vitamin E, C, B_6, and zinc.

- Check the expiration date. Multivitamins may not start smelling up the place after they expire, but they can lose their potency.

- Only take what is recommended. One a day is exactly what you should take. Don't double up on pills.

WHEN TO CALL YOUR DOCTOR

Sometimes if you're run down, you know the reason...you're stressed, or you haven't been sleeping enough, or you've been eating empty calories, or spending a lot of time around sick people. (New teachers notoriously catch many colds during their first year or two teaching.) This book suggests lifestyle changes for solving those problems and giving a hand to your immune system. But in some cases, if you're eating well, practicing good self care, and following the other strategies suggested in this book, but still feeling run down or staying sus-

ceptible to germs, there may be another underlying health problem such as anemia, a thyroid issue, or a sleep disorder such as sleep apnea.

See a doctor:

- If you have more than 4 to 5 colds a year

- If you have a chronic or ongoing infection

- If you have lymph glands that swell, even when you don't feel bad

- If you now have, or have ever had, cancer. Ask your doctor to check for signs of an impaired immune system.

SLEEP WELL, LIVE BETTER

If you're reading this book late at night, while you're feeling tired—put it down and go to bed! One of the best ways you can help your immune system is by getting enough sleep. In this chapter, we'll look at the reasons for getting enough sleep, as well as strategies for getting good, restful sleep.

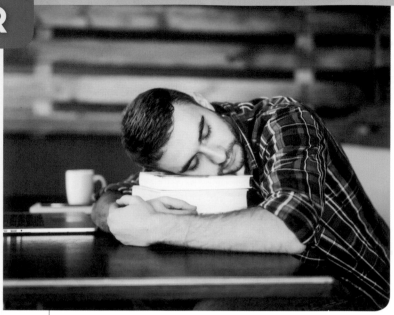

WHY DO WE SLEEP?

It should be obvious, right? Well it hasn't been so clear to some pretty smart people who have tried to figure it out. Here are some ideas that have been suggested over the years:

- Sleep is a response to boredom.
- Sleep occurs as a result of stomach vapors that cool the heart and block the brain's pores.
- Sleep is when the brain completely shuts down.

These and many other notions about why we sleep were proved wrong as researchers probed into the mysteries of sleep. Though many years of research have enlightened us to important aspects of sleep and why it's important, there is still much we don't know.

Here's a sampling of what we currently believe about why we sleep and about why sleep is so important:

- Sleep restores our mental energy. During dream sleep, we tend to store and reorganize information we have accumulated throughout the day. (The brain doesn't shut down after all!)

- Sleep is an important time when the body heals muscle tissue and restores itself. Our metabolic activity is at its lowest during deep sleep, providing an opportunity for the body to rebuild and heal. This is crucial both during the growth years of childhood and during adult life.

- During sleep, your brain waves slow down considerably compared to your waking state. This slowing of brain waves creates a combination of light and deep sleep that cycles repeatedly through the night. Your degree of refreshment the next day depends on how these cycles play out while you sleep.

THE COSTS OF TOO LITTLE SLEEP

The most obvious negative consequence of sleep deprivation is sleepiness. We all go through occasional periods when we get less sleep than we need. When we catch up on our sleep and return to getting the needed amount of rest each night, the sleepiness and fatigue disappear. But chronic sleep deprivation causes more than fatigue. It affects body, mind, and emotional balance.

Physical Effects

A number of experiments have been conducted to understand the long-term health effects of sleep deprivation. One high school student took the concept of adolescent late nights to the extreme by staying awake for 260 consecutive hours as part of a research experiment. While he lived to bask in the fame he had achieved, he has not recommended it to his friends. There appears to be no permanent physical impairment that results from sleep deprivation. But it does keep the body from performing the necessary tasks of renewing and healing muscle and nerve tissue that occur during sleep.

Another consequence of sleep deprivation is a compromised immune system. Even a modest reduction in sleep has been shown to affect immune response. If you are sleep deprived, you are at greater risk for flu, colds, and other infections. Fortunately, the immune system will bounce back quickly if you get the consistent rest you need.

Emotional Effects

If you have gone without sleep for any length of time, you know that you can become irritable, impatient, or even aggressive when you are tired. Some people have reported illusions and hallucinations when sleep-deprived. Even a small degree of sleep deprivation can contribute to depression or anxiety.

Mental-Functioning Effects

Anyone who has pulled an "all-nighter" studying for an exam or keeping a vigil at the hospital knows the muddled sensation of a tired mind. One of the immediate consequences of sleep deprivation is poor concentration and lack of sound judgment. Constant fatigue can also lead to memory loss or poor recall of known information.

Accidents

It should come as little surprise that a sleep-deprived person is also more prone to accidents. Perhaps the greatest danger is a sleep-deprived person operating heavy equipment or a motor vehicle. Research from the AAA Foundation for Traffic Safety shows that approximately 25 percent of subjects interviewed admit to falling asleep at the wheel of a car or truck at least once over the past year. Estimates of total crashes related to sleepy driving range from three to ten percent of all auto accidents.

DEVELOPING A RHYTHM

Years ago, before the invention of electricity, people went to bed shortly after the sun went down. Sure, it sounds boring, but there was a predictable rhythm to life that was dictated by sunshine and darkness. People worked hard during the day and slept well and long at night. But in modern times, we tend to move to a different beat. Our frenetic "always on the go" lifestyle has disrupted the rhythm of sleep that humans had grown accustomed to over centuries. Sleep now competes against work; personal, family, and social commitments; and a host of entertainment options, almost all of which are no longer restricted to daylight hours. This is not necessarily a bad turn of events, but it creates challenges for us in terms of getting the rest we need to stay healthy.

Fortunately, we have a built-in body clock that attempts to keep us in step with a normal 24-hour cycle of waking and sleeping. This body clock is often referred to as the circadian rhythm. The term circadian, translated from Latin, simply means "about a day." It is our body's natural way of trying to regulate not only our sleep patterns but a variety of other bodily processes, including digestion, elimination, growth, renewal of cells, and body temperature. When we work with our body's natural cycle, we can greatly improve not only our sleep but our overall health. When we fight against that cycle, on the other hand, our sleep, waking performance, and health can suffer.

Take, for example, a woman we'll call Diane. Diane is self-employed and works from home. She doesn't have a set time for going to bed or getting up each day; it pretty much depends on what she's doing on any particular day. She often works late into the night on various projects, finally retiring at 3 or 4 a.m. Following late-nighters, she tends to sleep in until about noon. Other nights she's so tired from her late-night routine that she goes to bed at 8 p.m. and sleeps for 12 hours. She finds that at least two or three days a week she needs a 30-minute "power nap" during the afternoon to get her through the day. Diane is wreaking havoc with her body clock with this inconsistent wake-sleep schedule. There is no rhythm to speak of. It's not surprising, then, that she often does not sleep well when she does hit the sack. She's not giving her body a chance to develop a predictable 24-hour rhythm that could better equip her for productive work during the day and restful sleep at night.

This is one of the main reasons sleep experts recommend going to bed and rising at the same time each day, even on weekends. It helps keep the circadian rhythm working in your favor. Different ages, sleep needs, and lifestyle patterns require different wake-sleep rhythms. The goal is to find what works best for you and stick with it.

AGE AND SLEEP

So far, our discussion has focused primarily on the sleep needs and patterns of average adults. For children, adolescents, and, to a lesser extent, seniors, these patterns and needs can be quite different.

Children

You may have noticed that infants sleep a lot—but not always at the times their parents want them to. During the first few months of life, an infant has two basic jobs: eating and sleeping. An infant typically sleeps an average of 16 to 18 hours each day and needs every bit of it for proper growth and development. Infants tend to sleep in four- to five-hour blocks of time and wake when they are hungry. The natural sleep-wake rhythm of infants is weighted heavily toward sleep. So in a 24-hour cycle, an infant will sleep two-thirds or more of that time. In contrast, an adult on average sleeps only one-third of that total daily cycle.

As a child develops, their sleep time gradually decreases. At six months, the average sleep time is 14 hours; at age two, that has dropped further to around 12.5 hours. By the time a child reaches age six, sleep time is reduced to about 11 hours, and naps are often no longer needed.

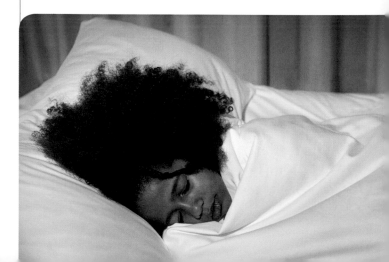

During a child's elementary school years, sleep patterns begin to resemble those of adults. Grade-schoolers sleep more deeply in certain phases of sleep, which indicates their brains are maturing in their ability to store and process information from the day.

Adolescents

Most teenagers have a love-hate relationship with sleep. They want to stay up way too late on school nights—or every night, in some instances. Then on a Saturday or a school holiday, they prefer to hibernate in bed for most of the day. It's not uncommon for a wary parent to sneak into their teen's room at 3:00 p.m. to listen for signs of breathing. While this pattern of sleep may be confusing to parents, there seem to be some good reasons for this erratic sleep behavior.

Research indicates that this tendency toward being a night owl may have a biological origin in adolescents. The bodily changes they experience in puberty may reset their sleep-wake clock so they are not ready to fall asleep until 11 p.m. or later. Of course, the problem is not so much with staying up late as it is with getting up early for school. The average teen needs about nine or ten hours of sleep a night, but few get that much on a regular basis. A teen who goes to bed at 11 p.m. would have to sleep until 8 or 9 a.m. to get their needed night's rest. But because they need to rise early for classes, most adolescents get seven hours or less of sleep a night. That's an average of two to three hours of missed sleep each night! The National Sleep Foundation reports that 60 percent of teens feel tired during the day and 15 percent report falling asleep in class during the past year.

Seniors

Answer true or false about the following statement: Seniors don't need as much sleep as they did when they were younger.

Most people would say "true." And most people would be wrong. It is a myth that seniors need less sleep simply because they are older. Older adults require the same six to nine hours of restful sleep as other adults. The stumbling blocks for seniors in getting this amount of sleep include poor lifestyle habits and chronic illness, both of which can disrupt sleep.

It used to be thought that the internal body clock of older people required them to get less sleep. Research has shown this notion to be false. It is true that seniors tend to rise earlier in the morning and become sleepy in the afternoon. This is due to the internal body clock setting itself to a different rhythm as we age. Social factors, such as going to bed early out of boredom, and medical illnesses and medications that cause fatigue and sleepiness, may also cause earlier bedtimes and early morning awakening.

WHY DO SOME PEOPLE SLEEP BETTER THAN OTHERS?

If you can stay awake for the answer, you'll discover that you're not alone in asking that question. It's estimated that over 100 million Americans are chronically sleep-deprived. There are two main reasons for this. The first reason involves lifestyle habits.

Lifestyle Habits

Ever since short-sleeper Thomas Edison invented the lightbulb, we have been staying up later into the night. But he doesn't deserve all of the blame. Over the years, we have evolved into a 24/7 culture that pushes limits. As work, family, entertainment, and a seemingly infinite number of responsibilities and experiences tug at our limited time, we tend to steal time from the most available source: our sleeping hours.

The National Sleep Foundation conducts a survey each year to measure sleep habits of Americans. Findings show that nearly two-thirds of adults do not get the recommended eight hours of sleep per night. Of course, some of these folks are short sleepers and don't need eight hours, but many do need that much and are not getting it. One-third of the respondents reported getting less than seven hours of sleep each night. And one-quarter claim that they are so sleepy during the day that their fatigue interferes with daily activities. The practical translation of these statistics: There are a lot of chronically tired people walking around. A common trick many use in an effort to catch up on their sleep is to spend more time sleeping on the weekends. While this may help somewhat in the short-term, it rarely balances the books. Instead, the sleep that is lost accumulates over time into what is called sleep debt.

You create a sleep debt when you "borrow" hours that you really need for sleep and use them for something else, often with the assumption that you'll try to "repay" them at a later time. Say, for example, that a fellow named John knows he functions best on eight hours of sleep. But he works two jobs and finds that he can't get everything done without staying up later at night. He averages about 6.5 hours of sleep a night. So the difference between the sleep he needs to be alert and fully rested and what he actually gets is 1.5 hours a night. By the end of the workweek, he has "borrowed" 7.5 hours from his sleep account (1.535 days). In an effort to make up for lost dozing time, he sleeps about nine hours each on Saturday and Sunday. So John makes a "deposit" of 2 hours back into his sleep account over the weekend. But this still leaves him short 5.5 hours for the week. So while a little extra sleep on the weekend helps, John never truly catches up on his sleep and feels chronically tired. He is tired so much of the time that he has begun to feel this is normal for him. The only way John can erase the debt is to change his sleep routine to get the sleep he needs on a regular basis.

Sleep Disorders

Those who are tired because of lifestyle habits tend to cheat themselves of sleep. But those who suffer from a sleep disorder feel they are being robbed of their sleep by a force beyond their control. Millions of people struggle with one of 80 known sleep disorders. People with chronic health problems (currently 45 percent of the population) are among those most prone to having a sleep disorder. The disruption in sleep may also be caused by pain, disability, medication, or other source.

When to Seek Help

You should seek medical help if your sleep problem persists for three weeks or more. Of course, if the problem is severe, it may be advisable to consult a physician sooner. For example, someone who gets fewer than three hours of sleep each night should not wait three weeks before seeing a doctor.

Problems with daytime sleepiness also demand attention. The most common cause of daytime sleepiness is not getting enough sleep at night. In this case, the first step may not be a trip to the doctor but an attempt to increase the amount of sleep you get at night. If you are still falling asleep or drifting off at inappropriate times (at work or when driving), seek medical attention as soon as possible. Such major daytime sleepiness is a serious symptom that should never be ignored.

If you decide to see a doctor, who should it be? Usually, it's reasonable to start with your family doctor. He or she will likely take a history of your sleep problem, conduct a physical exam, and order routine blood tests to rule out most medical problems. Should the results of these tests be negative, a referral to a sleep specialist may be the next step.

You should consider several factors when looking for a sleep specialist. First, make sure the doctor has the proper credentials. Sleep specialists should be board certified in sleep medicine. Sleep doctors often have training in a second area: psychiatry, neurology, or internal medicine.

If your doctor refers you to a sleep center for diagnosis, the center should be accredited by the American Academy of Sleep Medicine (AASM). The AASM is the professional organization for sleep medicine in the United States. Each accredited laboratory is inspected to ensure it meets standards set by the AASM. Sleep centers that are not accredited may or may not adhere to guidelines of the AASM. Be wary of a recommendation for sleep studies performed in the home. These tests have serious limitations and are often performed by those with inadequate training.

GET IT IN WRITING

By now, you may think you know whether you are getting enough sleep on a nightly basis. But consider these specific questions:

- How many hours of sleep do you average each night?
- How many hours do you think you need to function physically and mentally at your best?

- What is your sleep debt per week?
- How many times per night do you typically awaken from sleep?

Most people, when asked these questions, can only give approximate numbers. But the answers to these questions are very important for you to know if you want to correct current sleeping problems. The best way to begin is to keep what's known as a sleep diary.

	Time You Went to Bed	Time It Took You To Fall Asleep	Number of Awakenings per Night/ Reasons	How Long Awake Each Time	Time You Got Up in the Morning	Total Sleep Time	+/- Sleep Needed
Sunday							
Monday							
Tuesday							
Wednesday							
Thursday							
Friday							
Saturday							

A sleep diary will show you exactly what is occurring with your sleep habits. There are many variations of sleep diaries. Page 25 shows one simple format.

Virtually all sleep clinics instruct their patients to use sleep diaries at some point to gather important information about sleep habits before they begin treatment for problems. The answers you log in your sleep diary might surprise you! You might think you're getting eight hours of sleep, only for the diary to reveal that while you spend eight hours in bed, you only get seven hours of sleep because of bathroom breaks or other matters. That sleep debt accumulates quickly!

SETTING THE STAGE FOR BETTER SLEEP

Often, we are our own worst enemies when it comes to getting his needed sleep. Take the case of Henry. After racing all day at work, he continues his relentless pace into his non-work hours, trying to squeeze in all of the things he needs or wants to do. At some late hour he gets hit with fatigue. It's the first time since awakening early that morning that

he has even thought about sleep. And that's a major mistake. Because now, deciding it is time to go to bed, he assumes that putting a toothbrush in his mouth, peeling the covers back, and closing his eyes will perform a magical spell that will catapult him into deep, refreshing sleep.

But sound sleep is not what Henry typically experiences. After driving his body and mind at 80 miles per hour for the entire day and evening, he slams on the brakes and rolls into bed. While his intention is to sleep, his mind and body are not ready. He's taken no time or effort to prepare himself for a good night's sleep. But should he?

The answer is a definite yes, despite the fact that most people don't. That lack of preparation could have something to do with the fact that over half the population of the United States complains of sleep problems.

In order to maximize your sleep time, there are four main considerations. You must:

- Begin your preparations for sleep

during the day

- Schedule your sleep patterns deliberately
- Practice habits that help your body to relax before sleep
- Control your sleep environment

PREPARE FOR SLEEP ALL DAY

From the moment you wake up in the morning, you have choices to make that can affect how well you sleep that night. Making wise choices throughout the day can help you sleep soundly at night and awaken with renewed energy.

Exercise to Sleep Better

The majority of people claim that they don't exercise on a regular basis because they are too tired. Hmmm. Could that have something to do with sleep habits, perhaps? Chances are good that it does. If there were a competition to determine which lifestyle habit would win the title of "best intention never acted on," exercise would probably win. The reason we intend to exercise is that we all know how good it is for us. And research finds new benefits every day. As we discuss further in chapter 3,

THE EXERCISE-SLEEP CONNECTION

Everyone's body temperature naturally goes up slightly in the daytime and back down at night, reaching its low just before dawn. Decreasing body temperature seems to be a trigger, signaling the body that it's time to sleep. Vigorous exercise temporarily raises the body temperature as much as two degrees. Twenty or 30 minutes of aerobic exercise is sufficient to keep the body temperature at this higher level for a period of four to five hours, after which it drops lower than if you hadn't exercised. This lower body temperature is what helps you sleep better. So if you exercise five to six hours before going to bed, you will be attempting to sleep at the same time your temperature is beginning to go down.

That's the best way to maximize exercise's beneficial effects on sleep.

regular exercise improves heart health and blood pressure, builds bone and muscle, helps combat stress and muscle tension, and can even improve mood. Add one more benefit: sound sleep. Did you know that exercise can help you sleep sounder and longer and feel more awake during the day? It's true. But the key is found in the type of exercise you choose and the time you participate in it during the day.

What time of the day do you think exercise would best help you sleep? Morning? Afternoon? Evening? Right before bed?

Exercising vigorously right before bed or within about three hours of your bedtime can actually make it harder to fall asleep. This surprises many people; it's often thought that a good workout before bed helps you feel more tired. In actuality, vigorous exercise right before bed stimulates your heart, brain, and muscles—the opposite of what you want at bedtime. It also raises your body temperature right before bed, which, you'll soon discover, is not what you want.

Morning exercise can relieve stress and improve mood. These effects can indirectly improve sleep, no doubt. To get a more direct sleep-promoting benefit from morning exercise, however, you can couple it with exposure to outdoor light. Being exposed to natural light in the morning, whether you're exercising or not, can improve your sleep at night by reinforcing your body's sleep-wake cycle.

When it comes to having a direct effect on getting a good night's sleep, it's vigorous exercise in the late afternoon or early evening that appears most beneficial. That's because it raises your body temperature above normal a few hours before bed, allowing it to start falling just as you're getting ready for bed. This decrease in body temperature appears to be a trigger that helps ease you into sleep (see the sidebar on the previous page).

The type of vigorous workout we're talking about is a cardiovascular workout. That means you engage in some activity in which you keep your heart rate up and your muscles pumping continuously for at least 20 minutes.

Although strength-training, stretching, yoga, and other methods of exercise are beneficial, none match the sleep-enhancing benefits of cardiovascular exercise.

Try to schedule at least 20 minutes of vigorous exercise three or four times a week. Choose whatever activity you enjoy. Walk to and from work, or walk the dog. Jog, swim, bike, ski, jump rope, dance, or play tennis—just make it part of your routine. If you have any serious medical conditions, are very overweight, or haven't exercised in years, talk to your doctor about your plans for exercising before you begin. Be sure to start exercising slowly, gradually increasing your workout time and intensity, so you don't get sidelined by injury. Remember, regular exercise can help you feel, look, and sleep better.

Brighten Your Morning

Light tells the brain it is time to wake up. That's probably obvious to anyone who has had to turn on a light in the middle of the night and then has had trouble getting back to sleep. What may not be so obvious is that exposure to light at other times, particularly in the early morning, can actually help you sleep at night.

How does morning light improve sleep? The light helps to regulate your biological clock and keep it on track. This internal

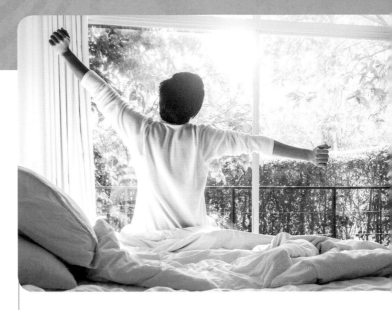

clock is located in the brain and keeps time not all that much differently from your wristwatch. There does, however, appear to be a kind of forward drift built into the brain. By staying up later and, more importantly, getting up later, you enforce that drift, which means you may find you have trouble getting to sleep and waking up when you need to. To counter this forward drift, you need to reset your clock each day, so that it stays compatible with the earth's 24-hour daily rhythm—and with your daily schedule. Exposing yourself to light in the morning appears to accomplish this resetting. Research has shown that people who are deprived of light for long periods of time (and so do not have their biological clocks reset) experience dramatic changes in their sleep, temperature, and hormone cycles. Although you probably won't be deprived of light for an extended period, getting less morning light than you need may make it more difficult for you to fall asleep and wake up at your preferred times.

Many factors can affect our biological clock, but light appears to be the most important. The timing of exposure is crucial; the body clock is most responsive to sunlight in the early morning, between 6:00 and 8:30 a.m. Exposure to sunlight later does not provide the same benefit. The type of light also matters, as does the length of exposure. Direct sunlight outdoors for at least one-half hour produces the most benefit. The indoor lighting in a typical home or office has little effect. Specially designed light boxes and visors that simulate sunlight are available. (They are often prescribed to treat seasonal affective disorder, or SAD, a form of depression that tends to occur seasonally, during the darker winter months.) Still, a half hour in front of even the most powerful light box does not provide as much phototherapy as does a half hour outside on even an overcast day—natural light is best.

Manage Stress

If you moved into a new neighborhood only to discover that it was plagued by smelly smoke from a nearby factory, you would likely be annoyed or angry at first. But after several weeks, you probably wouldn't notice it as much. You would become conditioned to the smell despite the fact that it may not be terribly healthy for you. A similar phenomenon can occur when we experience stress on an ongoing basis. We may be so bombarded with daily stress—in the form of hurried schedules, family commitments, traffic jams, and the like—that we become accustomed to it. We may not even realize how stressed we are until we're faced with a breakdown or an emergency—a "last straw." But such constant exposure to stress can make it difficult to get needed sleep and can compromise our overall health. For more about stress, see the next chapter.

Professional therapists who specialize in stress reduction will tell you that your body is the best guide to determining when you are feeling stressed. If you pay attention to how you feel both physically and emotionally, you can often intervene

Have you ever had to fight to keep your eyes open during a meeting or battled the head-nods while listening to a presentation? You probably attributed your desire to doze to the boring nature of the activity. But consider this: Children—who tend to get the amount of sleep their bodies need—don't get sleepy when faced with a boring situation; they get restless. So if sitting through a "sleeper of a speech" has you fighting to stay awake, consider it a hint from your body that you are not getting the sleep you need. This is especially vital when you are driving long distances. If you feel you have to turn up the radio or open a window just to stay awake during a "boring" drive, you are most likely too tired to be driving. The solution is not distraction but sleep.

before stress begins to interfere with your sleep.

What does stress management during the day have to do with sleeping well at night? Plenty. Have you ever had the unpleasant experience of crawling into bed exhausted, wanting to put a terrible day behind you, and spending the next few hours tossing and turning as you go over every detail of your day? That is stress at work on your mind. All of those emotions and thoughts throughout the day that were not dealt with at the time can work their way to the surface in the quiet of night.

In addition, the more you dwell on the upsetting events, the greater the effect on your body. When it senses stress, the brain sends a message to the body to release hormones that heighten alertness and prepare it for action. This is known as the fight-or-flight response. It's a beneficial reaction if you need to fight off a dog that threatens you on your walk or jump out of the way of a speeding vehicle. But when the stress is mental and there is no physical response necessary, that heightened state of alertness can keep you from relaxing enough to sleep. By learning to deal with stressors in your life more immediately during the day, you are less likely to be kept awake by them at night.

Nap Sparingly

Some people swear by naps; others find that napping during the day disrupts their sleep at night. Naps can be beneficial or detrimental, depending on how we use them. The urge to nap is greatest about eight hours after we awaken from a night's sleep. This is when our body temperature begins the first of two daily dips (the other, more dramatic dip, which we discussed earlier in this chapter, occurs at night). A short nap in the early to middle afternoon can bring a renewed sense of energy and alertness. A nap in the late-afternoon or early-evening, on the other hand, can disrupt your sleep cycle and make it difficult to fall asleep when you retire for the night.

To benefit most from a nap, take it no later than mid-afternoon and keep it under 30 minutes. If you nap for a longer period, your body lapses into a deeper phase of sleep, which can leave you feeling groggy when you awaken. If you are severely sleep-deprived and can't go on without a nap, it is better to sleep for a longer time to allow yourself to go through one complete sleep cycle. An average sleep cycle takes about 90 minutes in most people.

If you find you need a nap every day, take it at the same time so your body can develop a rhythm that incorporates the nap. If you try to take a nap but are unable to sleep, simply resting with your eyes closed may help restore some alertness and energy.

It's also possible to use naps to temper the negative effects of an anticipated sleep deficit. For instance, if you know you are going to be up late because of special plans, take a prolonged nap of two to three hours earlier in the day. This has been shown to reduce fatigue at the normal bedtime and improve alertness, although it may throw off your normal sleep rhythm temporarily.

Eat and Drink Wisely

How much of a direct effect diet has on sleep is still unclear. It's safe to say, though, that a balanced, varied diet full of fresh fruits, vegetables, whole grains, and low-fat protein sources can help your body function optimally and help ward off chronic conditions such as heart disease. Controlling portion sizes so you're taking in only enough calories to maintain a healthy weight can help keep diseases such as diabetes at bay. And since chronic diseases and the drugs required for them can interfere with sleep, eating wisely can help you safeguard your health and your sleep.

Adjusting your eating routine may also help you get a better night's sleep. Most people in this country eat a light breakfast, a moderate lunch, and a large meal in the evening. Yet leaving the largest meal to the end of the day may not be the best choice, since it can result in uncomfortable distention and possibly heartburn when you retire for the night. You might want to try reversing that pattern for a more sleep-friendly meal plan:

Eat a substantial breakfast. Because you are breaking your nighttime fast and consuming the nutrients you will need for energy throughout the morning, breakfast should be your largest meal of the day. Whole-grain breads and cereals, yogurt, and fruit are just a few examples of good breakfast choices.

Opt for a moderate lunch. Choose brown rice, pasta, or whole-grain bread and a serving of protein—fish, eggs, chicken, meat, or beans.

Finish with a light dinner. It is particularly important to eat lightly for your evening meal in order to prepare for a good night's sleep. Plan to finish your meal at least two hours before going to bed, preferably longer. If you need a little something to eat before you hit the sack, you'll find suggestions for late night snacks a bit later in this chapter.

In addition, you may want to try these tips:

- Reduce or eliminate caffeine, especially in the late afternoon and evening. Caffeine is a stimulant, which is why so many of us reach for that cup of coffee in the morning to get us going. And it's true that some individuals can drink caffeinated beverages all day long and still sleep soundly at night. But if you're having trouble sleeping, then limiting your caffeine intake should be one of the first steps you try to help improve your sleep. Be aware that coffee is not the only source of caffeine. Many sodas and teas, chocolate, and some medications, especially those for headaches, also contain caffeine. Check labels to help eliminate such sources of stimulation.

- Some people are sensitive to the flavor enhancer and preservative monosodium glutamate (MSG). In susceptible individuals, it can cause digestive upset, headaches, and other reactions that can interfere with sleep. MSG is found in some processed foods and in some Asian foods. Try avoiding foods that contain MSG to see if it helps you sleep better.

- Drink the majority of your fluids for the day by the end of dinner. A full bladder may be cutting into your sleep time. Drink plenty of water throughout the day. Water is essential to healthy bodily functions. Shoot for eight glasses, or two quarts, per day. But be sure to drink the majority of your fluids before dinnertime so you won't be making numerous trips to the bathroom during your sleeping hours.

- Skip the alcohol. Despite making you feel drowsy, alcohol may actually be disturbing your sleep.

SCHEDULE YOUR SLEEP

It might seem unnatural to schedule your sleep like you would an important appointment, but this is one of the most vital principles to getting a good night's rest. Here are several ideas for keeping a scheduled sleep routine.

Establish a Bedtime Ritual

Most of us begin our day with a morning routine. It helps us prepare ourselves physically and mentally for the day. So why not establish a bedtime routine that helps to prepare you for sleep? The purpose of a bedtime ritual is to send a signal to your body and mind that it's time to sleep.

You probably already have some regular bedtime habits, even if you haven't realized it. Brushing and flossing your teeth, lowering the thermostat, and setting your alarm clock may all be part of your evening routine. To help you get to sleep, you should perform these activities in the same manner and order every night.

Avoid activities that are stimulating or laden with emotion right before bedtime.

Starting to assemble your new computer or paying a stack of bills 30 minutes before bed would not be wise. Begin those types of activities earlier in the evening, and end them in time to go unhurriedly through your bedtime routine.

Establishing some type of bedtime ritual also provides closure to your day and allows you to go to bed and sleep with a more quiet body and mind.

WHAT'S YOUR RITUAL?

A bedtime ritual can be anything you want it to be as long as you do it each night. An appealing ritual for many might include: a light snack, laying clothes out for the next day, a warm bath or shower, brushing teeth, listening to soft music and/or reading, followed by lights out. Begin your ritual 30 to 60 minutes before your bedtime, and don't rush through it.

Stay Regular

Some people think going to bed on a schedule is only for children. While it's good for children to have a regular bedtime, it's also very good for adults who want to sleep like children when they hit the sack.

The idea is to go to bed and wake up at the same time each day, even on weekends. This regularity helps set your internal sleep-wake clock. Within weeks of keeping a regular sleep-wake schedule, you will begin to feel more alert than if you were keeping a variable sleep-wake routine. Not only will a stable rhythm of sleeping and waking improve the quality of your sleep, but it will probably also improve the quality of your life. Try it for six weeks and see the difference it makes in your energy and alertness.

EASE INTO SLEEP

Now that you know how to prepare for sleep during the day and schedule it at night, you're ready for bed. But before you peel those sheets back, consider how you might prepare your body and mind for that relaxing and peaceful sleep for which you long. The hour before bedtime is the most critical for good sleep. When used properly, the time right before bed can help you let go of the stressful, anxiety-provoking events of the day and promote a restful night's sleep. But if that last hour before slumber is not used properly, it can set the stage for a long night of tossing and turning. Try some of the following ideas to see which work best for you.

EARLY TO BED

There is nothing childish or old fashioned about going to bed early. Listen to what your body is telling you. If you find yourself yawning at 9 p.m., go to bed.

If you resist this urge even by 30 minutes you might miss the window in your sleep-wake cycle that could have put you into a deep sleep faster. Don't want to miss a favorite show? Use your DVR.

Seek Serenity

The key to preparing for sleep is to establish an atmosphere of peace and calm. Ease your mind and body with quiet yet pleasurable activities. You will create a sense of inner well-being that allows sleep to come quickly and easily. Most people find one of the following works well for them. Experiment with several if you're not sure.

- Read to relax. But choose your reading material with care. The idea is to read something light that won't stimulate your mind. In other words, you probably don't want to crack that new software manual. Better choices would be a popular magazine, a short story, or perhaps devotional reading.

- Listen to music. Choose music that relaxes you. In general, soft instrumental music has the most calming effect. Hard driving rock and pop beats often pull you into the music, causing you to be more awake, especially if the tunes are familiar. Another sound alternative might be playing a CD or mp3 of nature sounds.

- Try meditation or prayer. These activities, which help many people relax, can also help you be at peace with whatever is on your mind.

- Watch television, but only if it helps

you relax. Watching television is fine if you use some discipline. Falling asleep with the TV on is not the best way to start your sleep. In most cases, you have to awaken to turn it off, which forces you to have to fall asleep again. The idea is to stay asleep once you doze off. A better use of television is to watch it earlier in the evening and practice other relaxation techniques right before bed. If you must watch right before bed, don't watch in your bedroom.

Take a Warm Bath

One popular way to relax the body and slow down the mind is a warm bath, and you may find it fits the bill for you.

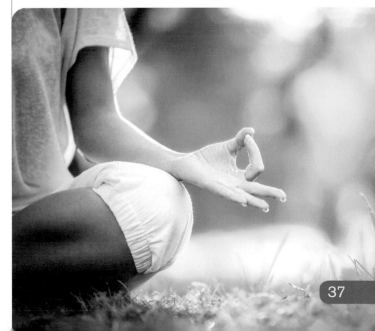

But you may want to do some experimenting with your timing. Some people find a nice hot bath just before bed makes them drowsy and ready to drop into sleep. If you do, enjoy. On the other hand, some people find that a hot bath is actually stimulating or that it makes them too uncomfortably warm when they slip into bed. If you find a just-before-bed bath makes it harder for you to fall asleep, consider taking the bath earlier, a couple of hours before bed. An earlier bath may enhance the gradual drop in body temperature that normally occurs at night and help trigger drowsiness.

RECIPE FOR A SOOTHING BATH

Why not make your bath as relaxing as possible? Try dimming the lights or using candles to create atmosphere. Play soft music in the background. Add two cups of Epsom salts to the bathwater to ease sore or tired muscles. Use a towel or waterproof pillow to support your head, and stretch out. Some people enjoy reading in the tub. But only read pleasurable material that you find relaxing.

Let It Go

You've just gotten off the phone with a relative who infuriates you every time you talk with them. Every single time they call, they launch into all the things they see wrong with the way you're living your life. Flying into your bedroom like a whirlwind, you try to get ready for bed. You're glowing with anger. You lie down on the bed and repeatedly slam your fist into your pillow as you try to find a comfortable position. But you can't fall asleep... you're on fire.

Too often people go to bed when their mind is a raging fury, agonizing over some event of the day. Don't make this mistake. You don't want your bed to be a place for anger or worry. Your bedroom should produce a feeling of peace and contentment.

When your emotions have boiled over, stay out of the bed and the bedroom until you cool down. Try journaling or writing your frustrations down on paper to help unburden your mind. Or try one of the relaxation techniques described in chapter 3 to unwind your tangled emotions. Once you've calmed down, then you can retreat to bed.

Make Your Bed a Haven

Most of us think of our bed as a place to sleep. But many people also use their bed for watching television, listening to the radio, talking on the telephone, eating, reading, or playing cards. If you really want to do all you can to sleep better, however, you shouldn't do any of these nonsleep activities in bed. When you do, the bed and bedroom can become associated with these activities rather than with sleep. Instead, you want to condition your mind and body to become drowsy and ready for sleep when you get into your bed, not ready and alert for a chat with a friend or a drama on TV.

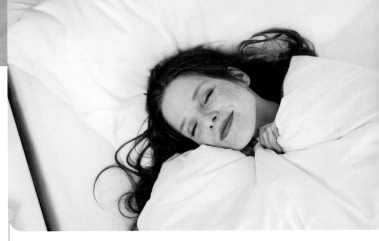

If you're one of those folks who sets the timer on the television or radio and drifts off listening to it, you might want to break yourself of the habit. You may not realize it, but you may be fighting off sleep just to hear the end of that monologue or the last bars of that favorite song. In addition, if you condition yourself to fall asleep only when you have that background noise, then if you wake up in the middle of the night, you may not be able to fall asleep without it. So you either struggle to fall back asleep without it or wake yourself up just to turn the device back on—neither of which is likely to improve your sleep overall.

Some people even go so far as to do work in bed. While this practice may help you catch up on paperwork, it can seriously disrupt your sleep. When you do work in bed, all of the associated stress becomes related to the bed and bedroom. Just getting into bed at night may subsequently cause your heart rate to increase, your muscles to tighten, and your thoughts to race. Whether you consciously realize it, the sheets, blankets, and pillows can become associated with your job, and their very sight and smell may cause thoughts of work to flood your mind as you try to fall asleep.

Stop Trying

While lying in bed, tossing and turning, you may become frustrated at your inability to slip into slumber, perhaps even repeating over and over, "I've got to go to sleep." The more you try to will yourself into sleep, the more conscious you become of not being able to doze off.

But sleep is unlike most activities in life. While trying harder is often the surest path to success in business, sports, or other waking activities, it is the surest path to failure when you want to sleep. Attempting to force yourself to sleep simply won't work. It only increases anxiety and tension. Sleep is most easily achieved in an atmosphere of total relaxation. Your mind should be empty of thought or turned to soothing and calming thoughts. Your body should be relaxed, your muscles free of tension.

If you find you can't fall asleep, the best solution is to get out of bed. That's right. Contrary to popular belief, the solution is not to stay in bed. If this happens with any frequency, and you do stay in bed, you may begin to associate your room and bed with feeling frustrated, uncomfortable, and unhappy. When you walk into your room, you'll immediately begin to worry about how long it will take to fall asleep. Consequently, it will take longer to drift off into slumber.

HIDE THE ALARM CLOCK

The bedside clock can be your number one enemy when you're having difficulty falling asleep. It acts as a constant reminder of how long it is taking you to fall to sleep and how little time you have left before needing to get up. It wakes you up just looking at it. So rather than letting it stare you in the face all night, set it for the waking time desired, then hide it away from your reach, or at least turn it around so you can't see the time.

Let your body associate any feelings of wakefulness with some other part of your home. Go to the kitchen for a drink of water. Go into another room and read, sew, draw. Almost any activity will do as long as it's calming, relaxing, and doesn't require intense concentration. Gradually, you'll become tired and bored. Usually, within 15 to 20 minutes, your body will be ready for you to try to sleep again.

Snack Lightly Before Bed

There's nothing like a grumbling stomach to keep you awake. So if hunger pangs strike as you're preparing for bed, have a light snack. Research indicates that a light snack can help you sleep more soundly. The emphasis, of course, is on light. Bedtime is no time to stuff yourself. An overly full belly can be just as detrimental to sleep as an empty one.

There are various theories about what you should have as a snack before bed. One age-old suggestion is warm milk. Some research has suggested that milk might be helpful because it contains tryptophan, a naturally occurring amino acid that the body uses to make serotonin; serotonin is a brain chemical that has a calming, sleep-promoting effect. Tryptophan is also found in a variety of other foods, such as turkey, tuna, peanuts, and cheese.

Other researchers emphasize the importance of eating a nighttime snack that is high in carbohydrates, such as bread, potatoes, cereal, or juice. The carbohydrates, they contend, help usher tryptophan into the brain, where it is then converted into serotonin.

Some sleep scientists recommend eating foods that are rich in magnesium and/or calcium. These minerals have a calming effect on the nervous system, and even a slight deficiency of them, they say, can affect sleep. Dairy foods are good sources of calcium. Sources of magnesium include fruits such as apples, apricots, avocados, bananas, and peaches; nuts; and whole-grain breads and cereals.

You might want to experiment with snacks from these various groups to see if they help you sleep. There's no guarantee they'll lead you to a good night's sleep, but you may find some of them helpful.

When choosing a snack before bed, another important point is that you should avoid foods that may promote heartburn, indigestion, gas, or other upsets. That means you should probably avoid greasy, fatty, and spicy foods. If you're lactose intolerant, skip the warm milk—or use a lactose-free variety. And if MSG causes you problems, don't treat yourself to those Chinese takeout leftovers.

Practice Relaxation Techniques

An excellent way to quiet your body and mind before bedtime is to use one of the active relaxation techniques such as progressive muscle relaxation, abdominal breathing, and visualization (page 59). These techniques help you to deliberately clear your mind of intrusive thoughts, wring the tension from your body, and put yourself into a peaceful state.

CONTROL YOUR SLEEP ENVIRONMENT

Some people can fall to sleep anywhere.

For most of us, though, our sleep environment has a substantial, if often overlooked, effect on our ability to get a good night's sleep. So let's take a look at how you can make your sleep environment more conducive to restful slumber.

Humidify Your Home

You're hot, and your throat is parched. Each swallow is agonizingly difficult. Your skin is dry and cracked, and your eyes are burning. All you can think of is a tall, cool glass of water. Where are you? The Sahara? Death Valley? The planet Venus? No, you're in bed in the typical North American home in winter, where the artificial heat that keeps us warm also dries out the air we breathe.

Although most of us prefer a temperature of 68 degrees or higher in the winter, we may pay a price for all that warmth. While heating systems warm our surroundings, they also remove a lot of moisture from the air. As you breathe this hot, dry air, water is also removed from your breathing passages, which can lead to throat or nasal discomfort or even upper airway infection. (Influenza viruses thrive in an atmosphere of low humidity.) If you

DOES COUNTING SHEEP WORK?

The oldest trick in the book may not be such a great trick after all. It was considered a given that the repetitive, monotonous activity of counting sheep would bore you to sleep. But a group of researchers at Oxford University recently decided to test that age-old theory. According to their results, counting sheep is actually so boring that it doesn't keep your attention long enough for you to relax your body and mind for sleep. What did seem to help the insomniacs to fall asleep an average of more than 20 minutes sooner was visualizing a relaxing, inviting scene. Check out our discussion of visualization on page 59 to learn more about this sleep-promoting technique.

ever feel the urge for a glass of water in the middle of the night to soothe a dry, parched throat, especially during the winter months, chances are good that dry air is a factor. Fortunately, there is a relatively simple solution to the dry air caused by indoor heating: a humidifier.

A humidifier adds moisture to the air, makes sleep easier, and provides a more comfortable and healthful environment. Humidifying your home can also ease some of your discomfort if you have a respiratory infection. If you are unable to afford

CLEAR BEDROOM CLUTTER

Is your bedroom a sleep sanctuary that feels calm, looks clean, and invites you to relax? Or does it have a computer, desk, files, and magazines strewn around, clothes on the floor, and books haphazardly stacked on your nightstand? To transform your bedroom into a restful sanctuary, start by cleaning. If your bedroom doubles as an office, move the equipment and related stuff to another location or hide it behind a folding screen. While you're in the mood, pitch or move all items out of the bedroom that might distract you from sleep. Then add subtle artwork, bedding, wall coverings, and window treatments that you find soothing.

a whole-house humidifier, get a portable room humidifier and keep it in the bedroom. Just be sure to clean the unit and replace the filter regularly, according to the manufacturer's instructions, to combat the growth of bacteria and mold.

Choose the Right Mattress

We spend about one-third of our lives asleep, and most of this time is spent on a mattress. Despite the amount of time we spend in bed, many of us ignore our mattress until the springs start poking us through the mattress pad. But a mattress has a lot to do with the quality of sleep and, therefore, with how we feel during the day. So give thought and attention to the type of mattress you use to ensure a good night's sleep and a well-rested feeling the following day.

Don't assume soft and fluffy is best. Poor support can lead to muscle stiffness as well as neck and back pain. Make sure your mattress isn't too soft and doesn't contain bumps, valleys, or depressions. Of course, too stiff isn't great, either. A mattress that is too hard can put pressure on the shoulders and hips. The ideal surface is gently supportive and firm,

DON'T FORGET THE CUSHIONING

The top layers of mattress cushioning are often what sell the customer. Comfort is what most people look for. But consider what the padding is made of. A cotton-polyester blend on top of polyurethane foam doesn't breathe well, yet this is the material used in many mattresses. Wool is a better material for layers closest to your body. Wool whisks moisture away from your body and keeps you dry while you sleep.

not rock hard or squishy. The mattress should mold to your body while still supporting it.

Keep in mind that mattresses don't last forever. Gradually, over time, they lose their firmness and support. The average life of a mattress is ten years, although most people keep them much longer. Once your mattress has developed lumps and sags, it is definitely time to replace it.

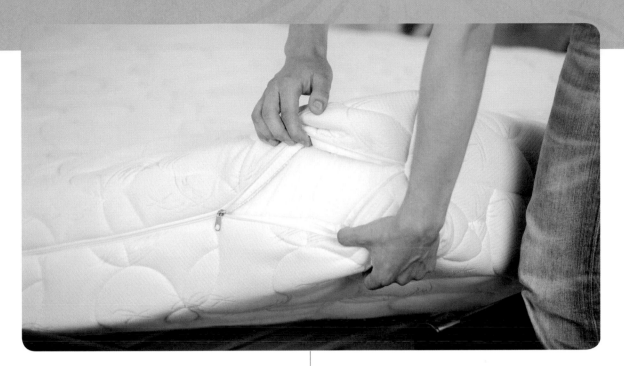

Mattresses come in different types. What are your options?

Polyurethane foam mattresses. These come in different degrees of firmness but often make people hot while sleeping. As you sleep, your body loses a pint or more of moisture per night. When a mattress doesn't "breathe" well or allow air to circulate, it can make you feel hot and sweaty.

Innerspring mattresses. These mattresses consist of rows of tempered steel coils layered between insulation and padding. Firmness and durability is based on the thickness of the wire and number of coils. The higher the coil count, the firmer the mattress.

Waterbeds. Waterbeds don't breathe, and they tend to sag under your body's heaviest parts. Some people love waterbeds and wouldn't sleep on anything else. But before you buy one, sleep on someone else's to see if it meets your expectations.

Most people choose innerspring mattresses because they offer many options for firmness, are cooler and drier because the air circulates around the coils, and are widely available.

Pick Your Pillow Wisely

Like the choice of a mattress, the choice of a pillow is a very personal matter. Although some people can sleep with their head on a block of wood, most of us are very particular about the type of pillow we use. Your head weighs more than ten pounds, so your pillow needs to provide you with support as well as comfort.

A good pillow supports you in just the right places. It should keep your head in line with your back and spine. But different sleeping positions require different pillows. If you tend to sleep on your side, you need a firm pillow that supports your head and neck. If you prefer sleeping on your back, a medium to firm pillow will offer you more cushion. Those who

sleep on their stomach should choose a soft pillow to ease strain on the neck.

Most pillows are made with synthetic fibers or foam, which are more friendly to allergy-prone people and easy to wash. If you must have a down or feather pillow, make sure it doesn't cause an allergic reaction in your sleep partner before you purchase it.

TEST YOUR PILLOW

If you're trying to determine whether your pillow is ready for replacement, try these tests. If you own a polyester pillow, fold it in half and place a shoe on top. If the pillow unfolds and knocks the shoe off, it is still good. If the shoe wins, the pillow probably needs replacing. If you have a feather pillow, fold it in half and squeeze out as much air as you can. (Leave the shoe out of this contest.) When you release the pillow, it should unfold on its own. If not, its goose is cooked and the pillow needs to be replaced.

Other types of pillows include orthopedic varieties that are designed to relieve pain and stiffness in the neck or back. Orthopedic pillows are more expensive than conventional pillows, but medical insurance may cover their purchase if your doctor prescribes them. You can purchase these pillows at a surgical supply store.

Also available are pillows designed to reduce or eliminate snoring. Despite the rather optimistic claims about these pillows, they are rarely effective. It's better to address the snoring problem directly with your doctor rather than muffle it with a futile search for the perfect pillow.

Most important, find a pillow that makes you feel comfortable. Just because your Aunt Gladys uses pillows made with hair from the East African two-humped camel, doesn't mean you should. And when your pillow starts to lose its shape or support, it's time to get a new one. Experiment with a variety of types, and stick with the one that provides you with the best night's sleep.

White-out the Noise

Our sleeping environment is rarely sound-free. It may be plagued by the chugging and whistles of trains, the roar of planes overhead, the clamber or loud music of neighbors, even the incessant cawing of crows in the early morning. The best solution, of course, is to eliminate the noise, but that's often easier said than done. So instead of trying to eliminate all nighttime noise pollution, try masking the noise with a white-noise machine.

White-noise machines are sound-producing devices. With the push of a button, a white-noise machine makes a soft, whooshing noise that can drown out many of the sudden and unpredictable noises that can disturb sleep. The white noise is easy to get used to and is actually quite soothing. More sophisticated models can produce the sounds of rain, wind, waves, or other nature sounds, although these may be too stimulating or distracting for some folks.

Unlike the television or a radio, the noise produced by a white-noise machine does not tend to awaken you from sleep because the volume is constant and the sound itself is unchanging. White-noise machines range in price from $50 to $150 and are available from specialty shops, mail-order catalogs, and even some department stores.

LIMIT THE LIGHT

Light tells your body it's time to wake up, so the darker your bedroom, the better. If an outdoor light shines into your room at night, purchase shades or curtains to block it out. Use a night-light, if necessary, but keep it away from your immediate sleeping area. When traveling, eye shades can be useful in shutting out unwanted light.

Put Pets in Their Place

In this country, pets are often considered part of the family. In many households, that means Fifi and/or Fido share their owner's bed. While this sleeping situation can be comforting to both human and pet, it can also disrupt sleep.

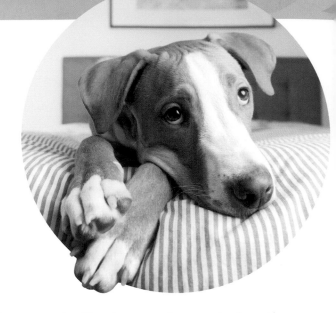

Some pets like to nuzzle up during the night. As you move, they move with you. By morning, you may find that you have been herded onto a tiny patch of the mattress while your pet has sprawled out freely on the rest. And, like people, pets change position various times throughout the night, which can awaken you. Add another person to the bed along with a pet or two and you have enough movement to simulate eight hours of earthquake aftershocks.

Then there are pets that wake their owners just for company. (Ever awoken to find one of your pet's favorite toys on your pillow?) If any of these scenarios sounds familiar, it's time to bar your pet from your bed. If you must, keep the

MAKE A SCENTED SLEEP PILLOW

Having a pleasant scent filling your nostrils when you get into bed may help you drift off to dreamland. A scented pillow is one way to create this effect. To make a scented pillow, you can, of course, spray a bit of essential oil onto your regular pillow. But you can also make an herb-filled sleep pillow by combining aromatic herbs and sewing them into a small piece of soft fabric. You'll want the pillow to be small and flat, so you can slip it into your regular pillowcase, on top of your regular pillow. Here's a sweet but potent mixture for an herbal pillow:

- 4 parts dried lavender leaves
- 2 parts dried hops
- 2 parts dried rose petals
- 1 part dried chamomile
- 1 part dried lemon balm

The herbs eventually lose their scent and should be replaced after about 9 to 12 months.

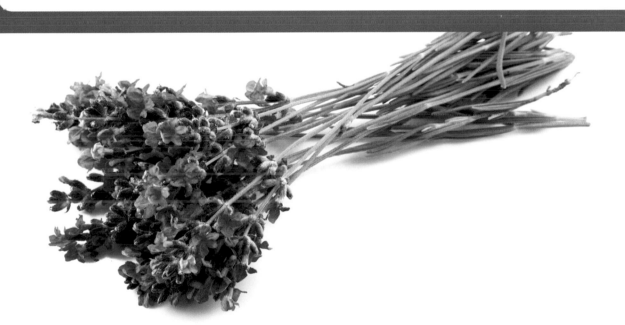

door to your bedroom closed when you sleep to keep your pet from wandering in. Moving your pet from the bed may be painful. You might even feel this is an act of betrayal. In truth, your pet will not love you less, but you will live together in greater peace and comfort. And you will get a better night's sleep.

HEALTHY MIND, HEALTHY BODY

If you've ever gotten a stress-induced headache before a big presentation, or woken up grumpy because you didn't get quite enough sleep, you already know: your body responds physically to your mental state of mind, and your mental state can be affected when you're physically hurt or even just run down. Our mind and body work together. There's even a fancy phrase in Latin to describe it: *Mens sana in corpore sano.* Whether you're in tip-top physical shape or suffering from an array of physical ailments, you can benefit from attending to your emotional, spiritual, and mental health.

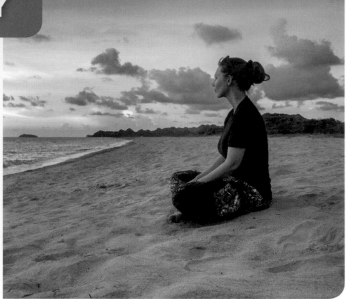

In this chapter, we'll examine some of the many ways you can boost your immune system with your mental state.

STRESS AND YOUR BODY

Stress can come from both positive and negative sources in your life—moving to a new house, having a baby, going through a divorce, grieving from a loss. When you encounter a source of stress, your body reacts physically. Some of those possible physical stress responses include:

- Muscle tension
- Changes in breathing patterns

The Roman poet Juvenal wrote in the late first century and early second century. His phrase, "*orandum est ut sit mens sana in corpore sano*" translates to, "You should pray for a healthy mind in a healthy body."

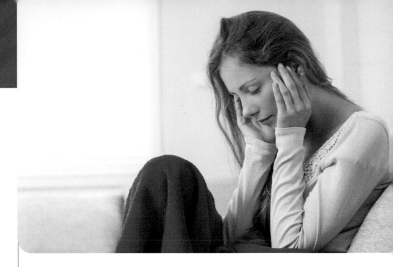

- Increased heart rate
- Increased blood pressure
- Release of stress hormones (adrenaline, noradrenaline, and cortisol)
- Heartburn
- "Butterflies" in your stomach
- Diarrhea
- Constipation
- Nausea

As unpleasant as some of these symptoms sound, they actually can be beneficial in the short term: faced with a threat, your body reacts by preparing for that threat, moving blood to vital systems in preparation for fight or flight. Over the longer term, however, these stress responses cause damage to the body, and affect almost every system. Over time, for example, muscle tension can lead to

Migraines and chronic headaches are linked to muscle tension—specifically, long-term muscle tension in the shoulders, neck, and head.

chronic pain in the musculoskeletal system. Chronic stress over time can lead to heightened blood pressure and inflammation in the circulatory system. Stress can affect blood glucose levels, especially in people who have diabetes or are at risk for it. Acid reflux can develop. Even menstruation and sexual desire can be affected.

MANAGING STRESS EFFECTIVELY

It's important to dispel the myth that you can avoid stress. If you breathe, you are going to encounter life situations that bring stress.

Some sources of stress are avoidable. If a friendship has become toxic over time, for instance, it may be time to let that friendship go. Even things that are good in and of themselves may cause unneeded stress; people can become overcommitted to the point where things that once brought them joy are now only another duty. In dealing with stress, the first step is often just acknowledging it: examining your life and thinking through what brings you happiness and what doesn't. Where are you in a rut?

However, we can't prevent all stress— and we wouldn't even want to! People who avoid stressful situations out of fear of them may actually increase their stress levels. Instead, we can work to acknowledge stress, address it, and process it in healthy ways. Let's look at some strategies for reducing stress.

DON'T FORGET TO BREATHE!

Have you ever noticed that when you are tense, you sometimes forget to breathe? When we are under stress, our muscles instinctively tense. Tight muscles, especially in the chest, shoulders, and abdomen, restrict the flow of oxygen into the lungs and make breathing more shallow. Shallow breathing allows less oxygen to reach the brain, which can actually decrease alertness and increase fatigue. The remedy: Remember to breathe.

One of the best things you can do when you're stressed is to take a few slow, deep breaths to bring more oxygen to your brain and help release those tight chest and abdominal muscles.

EXAMINE YOUR COMMITMENTS

Since you can't avoid stress, the best option is to learn to manage it. One key to managing stress is assessing what you have control over and what you don't. For instance, if your boss has set an unrealistic deadline for a project, you may have little or no control over changing that. But you do have control over how you respond to that deadline. And your response to a given situation is what you want to focus on as you seek to manage stress. You can choose to do certain things and not others. This ability to choose puts you in control and gives you the ability to make the situation work for you.

KEEP A JOURNAL

What stresses you out? What were the high points of your day? What were the low points? Daily journaling can help you

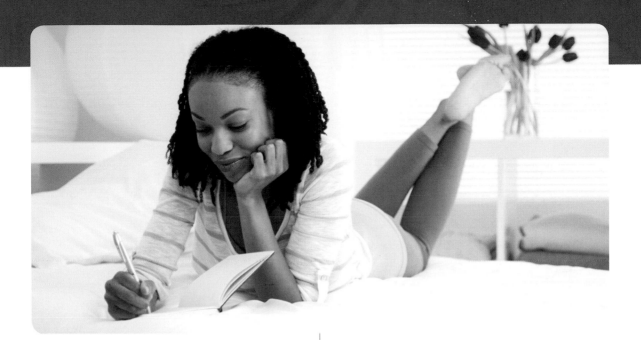

track the stressors in your day. Sometimes writing a problem down, getting it out of your head and onto paper, can help you see that problem more clearly. For recurring problems, you can also keep a "worry list." Write down a problem and the steps you're taking to handle it. If you find yourself dwelling on it, go to the worry list and put a check mark by it. Acknowledge the worry. Ask yourself if you have further information about the problem that would change your plan for dealing with it. If you don't, then tell yourself that you have noted it down, and direct your brain to focus on other things.

You can also include a "gratitude list" as part of your journal. See the next section for more about that!

PRACTICE GRATITUDE

Cultivating the habit of feeling and expressing gratitude can renew our appreciation for our family members, our friends, the beauty of nature, and so much more. It can deepen our relationships and bolster our mental, physical, and emotional health. Scientists at the University of Berkeley's Greater Good Science Center have found that making a daily list of three things you are grateful for works wonders. There is no need to go on a long silent retreat, when doing something as simple as focusing on a handful of things to be grateful for is enough to lower stress and make you smile more.

A University of North Carolina study tells us to think positive! The study looked at positive thoughts and attitudes as more than just being upbeat. It showed that being of a positive mindset actually adds value to life and helps you build skills like finding more options for a challenge, and seeing more possibilities to lead to a happier outcome.

Showing gratitude on a regular basis, such as weekly or daily, can have positive benefits on everything from achieving more goals, exercising more, and being more aware and alert, according to a series of studies done in 2003. Being grateful is something we can do at any time, but making it a regular practice is good for the body, mind, and spirit.

Here's one exercise to train you to practice gratitude: Before you rise to face the day, sit quietly for five minutes and think about someone in your life you are grateful for. Focus the mind on the feeling of gratitude, and the love you feel for this person. Breathe deeply, letting that sense of gratefulness expand like the ripples in a pond to everyone around you. Now, go face the day with a full heart and a happy spirit.

LAUGH IT OFF

What makes you laugh? Laughing is a tremendous way to let go of stress. When you laugh, your body produces natural painkillers and increases circulation. And just thinking about something funny can put stressful situations into proper perspective. So go on Youtube to find funny videos, rent a funny movie, or ask a friend to tell you a funny joke. If you're on Facebook or Twitter, ask your friends to share a funny moment, joke, or picture.

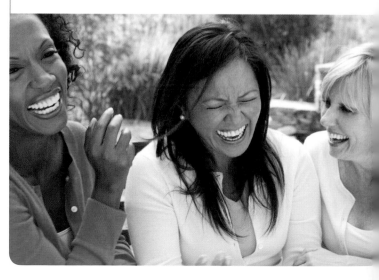

GIVE YOURSELF A BREAK

Even though you should not "run away" from your problems, a temporary reprieve can be very helpful. Immerse yourself in music. Take a vacation. Visit nature. Or just pamper yourself with a massage, aromatherapy, or an old-fashioned bubble bath.

SEEK A DIVERSION

Focus on a specific, enjoyable task that engages both your brain and your body. Hit baseballs in a batting cage. Learn how to knit or crochet. Do a jigsaw puzzle with your kids. Cook a meal. Take that class in painting, woodworking, or jewelry making that you've always been intrigued by. Many people have been enchanted by the trend in adult coloring books, which allows non-artists to relax and create something intricate and beautiful—if you haven't tried, check it out for yourself!

SET YOURSELF A CONCRETE TASK

Overwhelmed by your to-do list? Set it aside and do one, concrete task for a short period of time, maybe 10 or 30

10 WAYS TO LOWER STRESS IN FIVE MINUTES OR LESS

1. Sing a song. This helps with your breathing and channels nervous energy.
2. Wash your face and hands with a very hot washcloth.
3. Cup your hands under warm running water. Let it fill your hands and pour out.
4. Hug a partner, spouse, child, or friend.
5. Pet a cat or dog.
6. Hold your hands open, palms facing up, and focus on breathing slowly.
7. Run your hands along something with texture, such as fake fur or a textured carpeting. Focus on your hands and what they're feeling.
8. Drum your hands on a soft but resistant surface, such as a mattress.
9. Place your hands flat against the wall and push against it, as if you're holding the wall up.
10. Focus on your senses. What are you hearing? What are you seeing? What are you smelling? What are you touching?

minutes. For instance, wash dishes, clean a bathroom, weed your garden, or sort out a closet. Choose a task with strictly defined parameters, where you will see a visible change in a short period of time. This will boost your spirits—and give you more energy to tackle larger projects.

GET UP AND STRETCH

If your job requires you to work at a desk most of your day, take periodic breaks for your eyes and your muscles. Every 20 minutes or so, look away from your computer, blink several times, and look into the distance. Every hour or so, get up and stretch. Deliberately loosen the muscles in your shoulders and neck. If you have a longer lunch break, take a brisk 10-minute walk around your office or outside it.

CONNECT WITH OTHERS

Sometimes when people are stressed, they have the tendency to isolate themselves.

When we're going through busy periods, we can let our friendships fall by the wayside. But a quick conversation with a friend can actually boost our energy and leave us feeling restored. If you're feeling isolated or lonely, don't wait for a friend to call you—instead, reach out yourself. If you have a busy month ahead of you, try to book lunch with a friend in the middle of it, so you can have something to look forward to.

UNPLUG FOR AWHILE

Social media such as Facebook or Twitter can have a positive impact, connecting you to friends and relatives and introducing you to interesting ideas and funny jokes. But it can also be dispiriting, with a low signal to noise ratio. In polarized political times, social media can amplify outrage and anger. So give yourself a break from it—maybe make one evening a week "phone-free time," or make a rule that you don't check social media or e-mail after a certain hour in the evening. Put down your phone during family dinners, or while you're at a child's soccer or baseball game.

DO SOMETHING NICE

Sometimes, working to lift the spirits of others can have the unexpected bonus of lifting our own spirits. If you're down or stressed, look around to see what you can do for someone else. Here are just a few options:

- Send a funny or sweet "thinking of you" card to a friend.

- Donate to a charity or to an organization such as a museum or arboretum.

- Leave behind an outsize tip at your favorite restaurant.

- Pay a compliment to someone you know on their outfit.

- Express appreciation to a colleague for their hard work.

- Give flowers to your partner or spouse, a friend who's having a hard time, or a parent or child.

- Volunteering is a great way to put good in the world, especially if you're able to volunteer on a regular basis. Helping others and giving of yourself

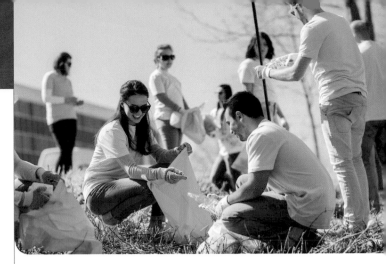

can give your spirits a real lift. It can also put your own issues in perspective and is a great way to refocus on things that are truly important in life.

DON'T PROCRASTINATE

Many of us are great procrastinators, living by the motto "Why do today what I can put off until tomorrow?" Would you consider yourself a procrastinator? If so, you can't afford to put off reading this section.

Putting work, projects, or tasks off almost always has bad consequences, one of which is increased stress. Getting your work done can be seen as another way of managing your stress. You can choose to put your time and energy into accomplishing what is before you and reap the benefits or put it off and worry about it. Tasks left undone can even intrude into your dreams at night and, in extreme cases, lead to nightmares.

Avoiding procrastination takes some discipline. There are certain techniques, however, that can help:

- Make a "to do" list for the day, then rank your list from most to least important. Start with the most important and work your way through them, checking each off as you complete it. If unexpected circumstances limit what you can accomplish that day, you will have put your limited time and energy toward the most important tasks. And this will leave you with a sense of accomplishment.

- Finish what you start. Leaving projects half-done is sometimes worse than not starting them at all. An incomplete job will occupy your mind

and make relaxing difficult. Also, work that is partly done robs you of the satisfaction that comes with closure.

- Keep promises to do tasks on time. Make schedules and stick with them. When promised work is late, it only becomes more difficult to face as time goes by.

- Learn to say "no." Sometimes we procrastinate because we feel overwhelmed by all of our commitments. Still, we continue to volunteer for tasks or projects because we don't want to tell someone "no." To combat this habit, make an effort to look realistically at your schedule and responsibilities before you commit to optional activities, and realize that knowing when to say "no" is better for your health than worrying about tasks you can't hope to accomplish.

With some planning and a little self-discipline, you may find it easier to relax at night.

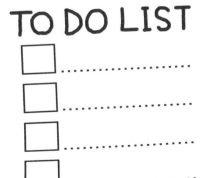

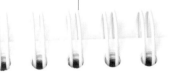

ACTIVELY RELAX

An excellent way to quiet your body and mind is to use one of the active relaxation techniques. These techniques help you to deliberately clear your mind of intrusive thoughts, wring the tension from your body, and put yourself into a peaceful state.

Progressive Muscle Relaxation (PMR)

When you tense a muscle for a few seconds, it naturally wants to relax. That is how PMR works. You start at your toes and deliberately tense one muscle group at a time, progressively working your way up the body. To prepare, lie on your back on the floor or on a couch or recliner in a room other than your bedroom. Begin by scrunching your toes as hard as you can for ten seconds, while keeping the rest of your body relaxed. Then relax your toes, and tighten and release your calf muscles, again leaving your other muscles relaxed. Then move on to your thigh muscles. Continue through the muscle groups of the buttocks, abdomen, chest, forearms, shoulders, neck and face. Take your time at it; performing the muscle relaxation one time, from toes to head, should take at least 20 minutes. By the time you work your way through the muscle groups, you should feel very relaxed. If you don't, repeat the entire cycle another time.

Abdominal Breathing

Rhythmic breathing is one of the best ways to help your body relax. There are many variations. This particular technique appears simple, but you'll need a little practice to do it properly. First, lie down on your back and begin to breathe normally. Now place your hand on your lower abdomen, just at your belt line, and slowly fill your lungs with air to the point that you can feel this portion of your abdomen rise. Take in as much air as you can and hold it for a couple of seconds. Then slowly release all the air in your lungs. Try to pay attention to nothing but the slow intake and release of air, the rhythmic rising and falling of your abdomen; don't rush. Repeat this eight to ten times.

Visualization

Imagine your favorite vacation spot. Maybe it's sitting on the sand with your

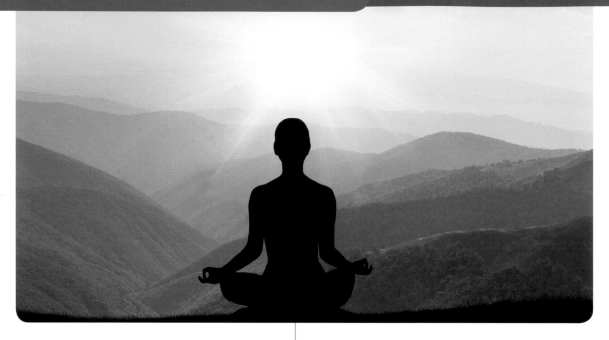

bare feet being massaged by the ocean surf, or scuba diving off some coral reef. Alternately, think of an activity you find especially relaxing: drawing, cooking, hiking, walking your dog, even shopping. The idea behind visualization is to use your imagination to envision something that tells your mind to enjoy itself instead of being focused on some worry or concern. It can be anything you find soothing. As you lie in bed, close your eyes and literally "go" to that place or "do" that activity in your mind. Chances are good that you will be feeling more relaxed in short order.

MINDFULNESS AND MEDITATION

Modern life seems to grow more hectic each day, and it's no surprise that people around the world have embraced mindfulness meditation. This technique sounds deceptively simple—"All I have to do is sit still?"—but requires practice, an open mind, and a quiet place to sit.

Much of what we think of as mindfulness originates in Hinduism and Buddhism, but the practice of meditation dates back millennia to the ancient religious beliefs of many groups. Contemplation is one of the human species' unique higher capacities, and even the word "mindfulness" evokes the awareness, abstract thinking, and inner world that the human brain enables us to have. What a biological novelty: to have such complex thinking that you need a way to quiet some of those thoughts!

Many spiritual traditions have some kind of altered consciousness, from the whirling dervishes of Sufi Islam to the glossolalia of Pentecostal Christianity. But mindfulness in the secular sense is not religious—it may be spiritual for you, and it's very personal, but no special belief or adherence is required. Rhythmic breathing and redirected thinking patterns, much like yoga, are suggested to reduce stress and anxiety. Think of it like an emergency dose of vitamin "calm."

Meditation is an excellent way to control troublesome thoughts and is a safe and simple way to balance your physical, emotional, and mental states. Meditation can help you pull your mind away from concerns about the past or future and focus on the present moment.

Meditation is not so much an emptying of the mind as it is a calming of the mind. One of the first things people realize when they begin meditating is how fast and furious their thoughts bombard them when they try to be still.

One novice meditator found this to be the case when he signed up for a local class on meditation. On the first night of instruction, he was told to lie on the floor and simply pay attention to his breathing for ten minutes. He thought to himself, "That's it? That'll be easy." He closed his eyes and, within seconds, it was like someone had pushed the play button on his mental DVR. Work hassles, bills, errands, plots from TV programs, and more

Heart disease is a major cause of death. But a 2012 study of people with coronary disease showed that taking a class in transcendental meditation reduced their risk of heart disease, stroke, and death by 48%. People who meditate have long said their practice keeps them healthy. Studies like this offer evidence of the powerful link between the mind and body.

ran through his mind like an old silent film set on fast-forward. By the time the ten minutes had elapsed, he felt more tense than when he started. But the experience gave him a clue about why he was having so much trouble falling asleep at night and why he felt so uptight and hurried all the time. After several weeks of participating in the class and practicing what he learned, he was gradually able to start roping in some of his worrisome thoughts and found that he could fall asleep much easier when he slipped into bed at night.

During meditation, the pulse rate slows, blood pressure falls, blood supply to the arms and legs increases, levels of stress hormones drop, and brain waves resemble a state of relaxation found in the early stages of sleep. These are all physical changes that can be brought about by learning to clear your mind of clutter and focus your thoughts. You can use meditation to clear and refresh your mind during the day or help you relax at night in preparation for sleep.

Although meditation sounds easy, it takes some practice to be most effective. Perhaps the hardest part is being able to block out intruding thoughts that threaten the peacefulness you seek. But if you practice every day, it will become easier, and you're likely to find that you look forward to these respites from your busy life.

Being mindful means being completely present to the feelings, sensations, and experiences of the moment. It means putting away watches and phones and devices and tuning into nature or the sound of your own breath. It means having no sense of worry, need, fear, demand, or expectation of what should be and instead allowing life to unfold as is. Mindfulness requires no equipment or membership.

You only need:

- A quiet place free from interruptions
- Music, a guided meditation, or pure silence
- The ability to sit still for at least ten minutes
- To experience what is, without resistance

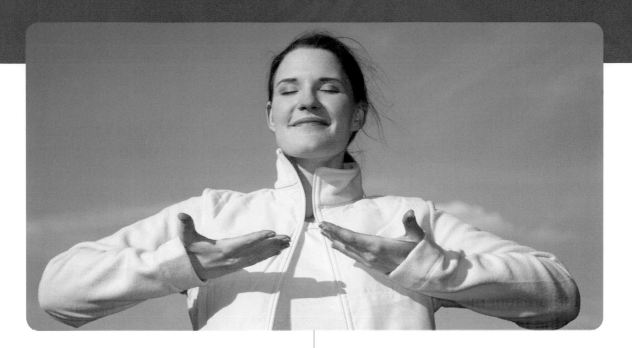

- Patience to focus and center your breathing
- The desire to live a more balanced, harmonious life

Exercise #1

Despite a popular myth, you don't need to contort your body into a cross-legged lotus position to meditate. A sitting or lying position will do just fine. (If you choose a sitting position, keep your spine straight but your shoulders relaxed.) It also helps to have a quiet place where you won't be distracted or disturbed. Once you're situated, close your eyes and breathe slowly, feeling the air enter your lungs. Next, exhale slowly, feeling the air leave your body. Keep the focus on your breathing. If your mind wanders off, gently bring your focus back to your breathing. You want your attention to remain on your breathing to keep you in the present moment. This way you won't be distracted by past or future events that may carry your mind away and possibly bring anxiety.

Practice this for 15 minutes each day. It can be especially helpful right before bed if you notice your mind is racing.

Exercise #2

Close your eyes now and repeat to yourself: "I am here, now. I am here, now." Allow the chaos of the day to drift away on the ocean of your conscious awareness.

"I am here, now." Let go of what weighs you down in body and in spirit. "I am here, now." Be here, now.

Exercise #3

As soon as you notice you are worrying about the future, or regretting the past, quiet your mind and bring it back to the present moment. Allow the feeling of calmness and clarity to wash over you. Breathe in the "now" and breathe out any concerns of "then." Centered, continue with your day.

Exercise #4

The breath is your healing power. Breathe in the white healing light. Let it wash over the unwellness in your body, restoring it to balance. Exhale illness and inhale strength. With each new breath, feel yourself empowered and renewed. Let the rhythm of your breathing be like the ocean waves, taking out sickness, bringing in wholeness.

Exercise #5

What makes you happy? Envision one thing that brings you joy and let that be the focus of your meditation today. Free the mind of everything but the love you feel, whether for a person, place, or object. Immerse yourself in appreciation and gratitude for this beloved presence. This simple practice opens the heart to the wonders of your daily life.

Exercise #6

How often do you stop and think about what you're thinking? Slow down and quiet the mind. Observe the thoughts that move in and out of your mind. Are they mostly negative? Positive? Empowering, or disempowering? Meditation allows you to become aware of your mind chatter and ultimately think better, clearer, more healthy thoughts.

Exercise #7

Visualize a lovely bench at the edge of a field of wildflowers. Sit down, in your mind, and look at the colors spread across the field like a painter's palette. Feel the sun and the breeze and relax, basking in the warmth and beauty of nature. Listen to birds in the trees bordering the field. Stay here awhile, among the flowers, among the birds.

Exercise #8

My mind is like a jar of water, pouring out, emptying into the greater sea of consciousness. Now empty, I fill my mind with light. I let the light overflow and expand outward, glowing, warming. I focus on the light and let myself bask in the glow of pure love and positive energy. My mind becomes the light.

Exercise #9

I am formless. I am energy. I am light. I am vibration. I breathe in the energies of peace and harmony. I breathe out the energies of anger and fear. I become lighter with each breath, in and out, calming and expelling. I become free with each pass of air into my lungs, letting go of my burdens and cares. I am formless, boundless energy.

Exercise #10

Pausing in the rushing and chaos of my day, I stop and breathe deeply. Closing my eyes, I bring my focus into the present, mindful of exactly where I am in this moment. Here, I rest for a while, just breathing. I am totally present and aware of my surroundings. My focus is laser sharp and my mind is clear. From this place of presence, I finish my day with clarity and calm.

Exercise #11

Meditation can help lessen pain. Focusing on the breath, or a mantra, helps keep the mind occupied and the body relaxed. Imagine white, healing light moving over the painful area. Feel it permeate every cell of the body. Breathe into the pain and embrace the light, then breathe out the pain, letting only light remain.

Exercise #12

Energy is life. During meditation, imagine you are nothing but vibrating waves of energy. Visualize your vibration rising higher. Give it a light and vivid color and a positive sensation. Experience the life energy moving through your body, lifting each cell into a vibration of healing and wholeness. Let your heart match the frequency of joy.

Exercise #13

Notice a flower in bloom as you go about your day, or picture one in your mind. Look closely at the intricacy of the petals. Imagine scents that soothe the mind and delight the soul. Remember peaceful walks in parks and gardens. We are nourished by the sun's warm rays. We raise our faces toward the sky.

Exercise #14

Vital energy flows through me as I sit in stillness. My mind calms and I am in tune with the vibration of the energy within. I let this energy expand outward, creating an aura of abundance, joy, and happiness that affects those I come in contact with. I am vibrant with the life force. I radiate rays of love.

Exercise #15

Visualize a beautiful beach. The air is warm, the sand white and clean. Listen to the rush of the waves and the call of gulls flying overhead. Children laugh as they run past. Feel the sun's rays on your skin. Taste sea salt upon your lips as time slows down. The cool breeze rustles your hair. You are relaxed, completely at peace.

ACUPUNCTURE AND ACUPRESSURE

Acupuncture dates back thousands of years and is rooted in Eastern healing practices. It's based on a concept that all disease is the result of an imbalance of subtle energy moving throughout the body. This energy moves along 14 pathways in the body called meridians. Through the ages, practitioners have identified and charted these meridians. Treatment by an acupuncturist involves inserting very fine needles at various points along these meridians to increase, decrease, or balance the energy flow.

In the Western scientific community, there is a great deal of skepticism about the use of acupuncture, mainly because there have not been a lot of well-designed, well-controlled studies proving its effectiveness. The National Institutes of Health, however, has stated that there is enough evidence to indicate that acupuncture can be helpful in controlling nausea and certain types of pain. Acupuncture has also been suggested—and in the East, used—as a remedy for insomnia, although scientific proof of this particular benefit is lacking. Still, acupuncture might be worth a try, especially for people suffering from chronic pain.

Most people have heard about someone who has been helped by acupuncture but are reluctant to try it themselves because they fear having needles inserted into their body. But the consensus of most people who have used acupuncture is that the procedure causes little or no discomfort, and many swear by the benefits they've received. Side effects from acupuncture are also rare and appear to result mostly from treatment by unqualified practitioners.

If you decide to try acupuncture, seek out a licensed practitioner, if your state governs this profession, or one certified by the National Commission for the Certification of Acupuncturists. In addition, check to be sure the acupuncturist uses

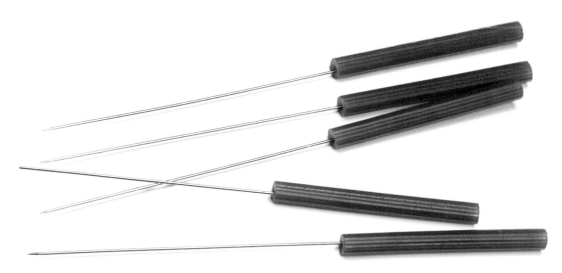

sterile, disposable needles, to decrease any risk of transmission of blood-borne infectious organisms.

A close cousin of acupuncture is acupressure. Acupressure relies on the same meridian points as acupuncture, but finger pressure, rather than a needle, is used to stimulate points along the meridians to increase, decrease, or balance the energy running through the body.

AROMATHERAPY

Aromatherapy is the therapeutic use of essential oils to comfort and heal, and it is one of the fastest growing complementary therapies in the Western world. In aromatherapy, the essential oils are used topically rather than taken internally. The essential oils are said to stimulate an area of the brain, known as the limbic system, that controls mood and emotion. Solid scientific backing for aromatherapy is lacking, but there's no doubt that many people find it a soothing complement to other self-help measures to ease tension, promote relaxation, and aid in sleep. So you may want to give it a try.

CALMING ESSENTIAL OILS

- Bergamot
- Chamomile
- Clary sage
- Lavender
- Lemon balm
- Orange
- Rose
- Sandalwood
- Sweet marjoram
- Ylang-ylang

You can try using essential oils singly or in combination. The essential oils are generally available at health food stores, although these days many drugstores also carry a variety of the oils.

Try adding a few drops of essential oil to warm water for a relaxing bath or foot-bath, or spritz the oil onto a handkerchief or small pillow. You can also apply a few drops to a heat diffuser near your bed to spread the scent through the room or use a specially made ring that can be placed on the lightbulb of a bedside lamp; the heat of the bulb diffuses the scent.

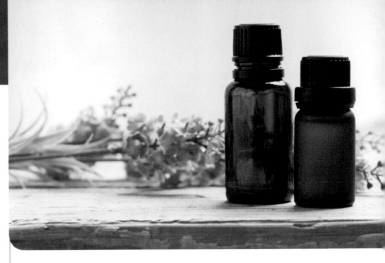

You might also want to try combining the relaxing benefits of aromatherapy and massage by creating your own scented massage oil. Dilute one to three drops of essential oil per teaspoon of an un-scented carrier oil, such as almond or grape-seed oil. (Do not apply undiluted essential oil directly to your skin.) Since some people are more sensitive to the oils than others, start with the smallest amount, and experiment until you find the combination that works best for you.

BIOFEEDBACK

Biofeedback training can help you learn to consciously control certain physical responses to stress. It begins with the use of a simple electronic device that monitors your heart rate, breathing, blood pressure, and/or muscle tension through electrodes that are placed on your skin. These electrodes give "feedback" about what your body is doing under certain conditions. You can then use this feed-back to retrain your responses.

For instance, when you are in a stress-ful situation—or even when you are just thinking about one—your heart rate tends to speed up, your breathing quickens, your blood pressure increases, and your muscles tense up. Conversely, by shift-ing your thoughts to calming scenes or situations or by consciously taking slow, deep breaths, you can slow your heart rate, lower your blood pressure, and ease muscle tension. The biofeedback machine makes these reactions easier to recognize. For example, the machine may be set to beep at every heartbeat, so you can hear when your heart is racing or when it's slowing. The combination of this feedback with training in relaxation techniques, such as visualization, medita-tion, or even simple breathing exercises, can thus help you to notice when stress is negatively affecting your body and ac-tively take steps to reverse those effects. With practice, you become better able to recognize stress responses so that eventually you no longer need the biofeedback machine. In this way, biofeedback can help individuals with poor stress management, anxiety, or obsessive thoughts.

Most people who decide to try biofeedback visit a clinic where a trained professional in biofeedback can guide them through the process. If you take this route, look for a biofeedback practitioner who is certified by the Biofeedback Certification Institute of America. The option of purchasing inexpensive biofeedback equipment to use on your own is also available. These home units typically come with detailed instructions for proper use.

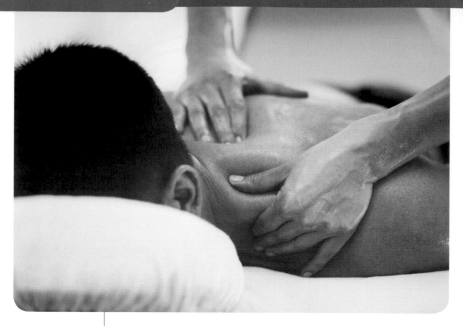

GET A MASSAGE

Massage is one of several hands-on strategies known collectively as body-work. And if you've ever had a good, thorough massage, you know the feeling of being "worked over." But you also know how relaxing it can be.

Massage and Pain Relief

Many types of pain have reportedly responded to massage therapy. These include back pain, pain from cancer and cancer treatment, carpal tunnel syndrome, fibromyalgia, migraine, muscle strain, neck pain, rheumatoid arthritis, temporomandibular joint disorder (TMD), tension headache, and whiplash. Massage may also play a role in the prevention of pain. For example, massage can soothe away tension before it triggers a headache, while a post-workout massage may help reduce an athlete's chances of getting sore muscles later on. In addition, massage helps relieve stress, anxiety, and depression, whether these result from illness, injury, trauma, or

HOMEMADE MASSAGE OIL

Oil allows your hands to move freely over the body during massage. While a variety of massage oils are on the market, you can also make your own. Choose a vegetable-based oil that has little or no scent of its own. Almond oil is a good choice because it is light and odorless. Avoid olive oil, which is too heavy and pungent. Then, to enhance the experience, you can add a few drops of an aromatic essential oil, such as lavender or chamomile, both of which tend to have a relaxing effect.

life's everyday pressures. If you have high blood pressure and have been told you need to relax more, getting regular massages may be a tool you can add to your kit.

How does massage work to relieve pain? One theory is that the pressure from massage closes down the pain gate to the brain, so the pain signals sent by your muscles aren't perceived by your brain. Massage also seems to relax muscular tensions that can trigger pain. And it may improve circulation, reduce stress hormones such as cortisol and nor-epinephrine, and stimulate the flow of body chemicals that serve as natural painkillers and

mood-elevators. People also report that massage helps raise their energy levels and get better, deeper sleep.

You might want to spring for a massage from a professional. One session may be all it takes to get you hooked. If you do opt for a professional massage, be sure to tell the practitioner if you have any particular illness or injury that they should be aware of, such as arthritis or fibromyalgia.

One of the good things about massage, of course, is that you don't have to visit a professional to capture its benefits. You can ask your partner, friend, or family member for a soothing rubdown. You can also give yourself a mini massage, focusing on the muscle groups that are within reach. Using small, circular movements with your fingers and hands, you can massage your scalp, forehead, face, neck and upper shoulders, lower back, arms, legs, and feet. There are also a variety of massaging devices available in various price ranges that can help extend your reach or provide soothing heat as well as relaxing vibrations.

History of Massage

Humans in diverse cultures have used massage for thousands of years as a means to improve health. The ancient Egyptians treated diseases with massage, and for centuries the Chinese have considered massage to be an essential ingredient of their approach to health care.

Modern massage was introduced to the United States in the 1850s by two New York physicians who had studied in Sweden. The first massage therapy clinics were opened here after the Civil War by two men from Sweden. Massage became popular for a while during the 1870s, but public interest gradually faded. Today, however, many doctors

WHEN MASSAGE ISN'T A GOOD IDEA

Massage should never be applied to the site of an open wound, injury, cancer, or skin infection. People with a history of blood clots should avoid deep, high-pressure massage techniques that might loosen a blood clot and lead to an embolism. If you have any doubts about whether you have a health condition that would contraindicate massage therapy, talk to your primary health care provider.

advocate the value of massage as useful therapy for many conditions.

Types of Massage

Generally defined, massage is the kneading, stroking, and manipulation of the soft tissues of the body—that is, the skin, muscles, tendons, and ligaments. One question that people have is whether massage will cause pain. It's true that sometimes muscles will ache as they're massaged and tension is worked out, but don't be pressured into a massage that's too intense by thinking, "no pain, no gain." You may also experience some soreness the day afterward, as if you've been working out. Ice can help, as can gentle stretching.

There are dozens of different massage techniques. Here are some of the more common.

Swedish massage. Stroking, kneading, and mild tapping of soft tissues are all part of Swedish massage, which is the most frequently used type of massage in the United States. The therapist uses oil or lotion so his or her hands can move smoothly over the skin. In general, if a spa, gym, or clinic is offering "massage," they're referring to Swedish massage. They're often offered in blocks of 30, 60, or 90 minutes.

Deep-tissue massage. This technique, similar to Swedish massage, utilizes deeper pressure in order to loosen tight muscles. It's considered especially useful for treating chronic conditions. People frequently feel sore after deep-tissue massage, and if you have arthritis or a similar condition, check with your doctor before committing to deep-tissue massage—it may not be the type of massage that's best for you.

Chair massage. You'll see these massages offered in places like airports or hotels. These massages can be a quick way to relieve some stress if you have 20 minutes to spare.

Amna and shiatsu. Amna is traditional Japanese massage, based on Chinese Traditional Medicine. Modern shiatsu, in turn, developed from amna. The term "shiatsu" means "finger pressure," and as with acupressure, fingers and palms are used extensively to manipulate the muscles. Shiatsu is a bit different from the Swedish massage that most Westerners are used to. There is no use of oil, so people do not generally disrobe; it's customary to wear loose, comfortable clothing to a shiatsu massage.

Hot stone massage. Hot stone massage involves placing smooth stones warmed by water on specific points on the body; the heat acts to relax the muscles. Cool stones can sometimes be used for contrast. The massage therapist may also hold the stones and use them to apply pressure.

Prenatal massage. Prenatal massage can help expectant mothers relieve aches and pains caused by pregnancy. Therapists work with their clients in order to make them comfortable and use positions that are safe for mother and baby. Women with high-risk pregnancies should, however, consult their doctor or midwife before beginning a massage program.

Geriatric massage. Massage can be very helpful for older patients, especially those who suffer from common conditions like high blood pressure or arthritis. In general, the practitioner will use a lighter, gentler touch for older clients.

Reflexology. Reflexology is massage that focuses on the feet, although the hands are sometimes also involved. Specific points on the feet and hands are thought to be reflex areas for other parts of the body, including the glands and organs. The therapist applies pressure

to these spots, both to diagnose what's wrong and to stimulate healing of the corresponding body part.

Sports massage. Specifically tailored for the athlete, sports massage focuses on parts of the body that get frequent use in a particular sport. For example, the legs of a cyclist and the arms of a swimmer get special attention. Massage before athletic activity helps warm up the muscles, while a post-workout massage seems to stimulate blood circulation and clear away lactic acid residues that cause muscle soreness.

Thai massage. A Thai massage therapist not only applies pressure to various parts of the body, but stretches the body. A Thai massage can look a bit like someone helping someone else achieve a yoga pose! It's meant to increase flexibility and range of motion. Wear loose, comfortable clothing to a Thai massage.

Trigger-point therapy. Trigger points are sensitive spots in the muscles that are often painful. They result from repetitive motions, injuries, accidents, or other types of trauma. Over time, disease and aging can increase the painfulness of sensitive trigger points. Deep pressure applied to these areas brings about pain relief. For chronically irritable trigger points, several sessions may be needed to completely clear the problem.

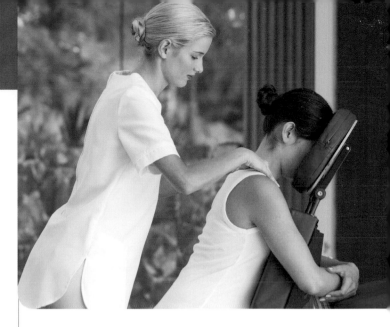

Finding a Massage Therapist

You can often find a massage therapist through referrals from friends or health care providers, or by reviews on Yelp or similar web sites. You can also check the web site for the American Massage Therapy Association (amtamassage.org)

Before an appointment, confirm that your prospective massage therapist is licensed to practice in your state and does the type of massage you're interested in. (Most, though not all, states regulate massage therapists.) If you're not sure what type of massage would be right for you, talk about any problems you're having, any health conditions you have, and what your goals are in order to get guidance. If you're getting a massage at the recommendation of your doctor or after an injury, check your insurance to see if they cover massage therapy (and what limits apply) and check with the clinic or spa to confirm that they take your insurance. Ask them if there are any forms you will need to fill out, or that you should fill out in advance—many clinics will have an intake form asking about your general health, any medications you're on, and so forth.

You may also want to ask beforehand

> ### FOOD AND DRINK
>
> In general, it's recommended that you don't eat heavily before a massage. Do, however, stay hydrated, both before and after your massage. Many massage therapists will offer you a glass of water after your session as a standard practice.

about tipping guidelines—in the U.S., it's generally customary to tip in spa settings, but not always when you're going through a medical practice.

At the session itself, discuss the problems you want to alleviate and what areas of the body you'd like the therapist to focus on. A good massage therapist will work with you to make the experience comfortable, productive, and relaxing. Throughout the massage, the massage therapist will probably check in with you on your comfort level. Don't be afraid to ask questions or to check in with the therapist if something feels wrong or even just less than optimal. Here are some things to consider:

- Would you like more or less pressure to be applied?

- Are you experiencing unexpected pain?

- In a hot stone massage, are the stones too hot for comfort?

- Is the room too warm or too cold?

- If music is playing, is it too loud or distracting?

- Do you have any scent allergies or

sensitivities that mean that certain oils or lotions are not for you?

With some types of massage therapy, such as Swedish massage, it's usual to disrobe to some level so that oil can be applied. The therapist should respect your comfort level, leaving you alone to remove clothing and, throughout the session, draping a sheet or cover over the parts of the body that aren't being worked on.

A therapist who pushes you to disrobe further than your comfort level, who doesn't listen to your needs, or who talks during the session if you ask for silence, is not the massage therapist for you! Don't be afraid to speak up yourself if something seems off!

GET MOVING

Today, many of us lead a lifestyle that's more sedentary than that of our ancestors. That lack of exercise can have serious consequences—we need exercise to keep our heart, muscles, and lungs healthy. Study after study shows that regular exercise can reduce the risk of heart attack and stroke, help people manage conditions such as prediabetes and diabetes, and even play a part in maintaining good mental health.

From the Ancient Texts

In traditional Chinese medicine, there is an understanding that too little exercise can lead to stagnation of qui and blood, and subsequently, a variety of diseases. Some of the traditional Chinese ideas about lack of exercise are expressed in the ancient texts:

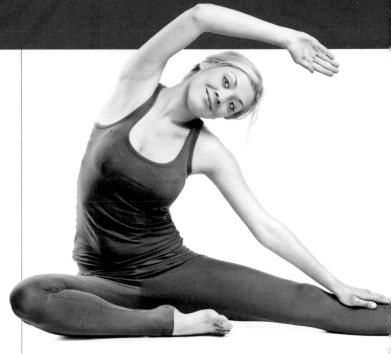

- "Sleeping or lying down too much hurts the qi." When a person over-sleeps, he or she typically feels tired all day.

- "Too much sitting hurts the muscles." This refers to the fact that lack of exercise causes the muscles to atrophy.

- "A running stream doesn't go bad." Stagnant water easily becomes spoiled; stagnant blood and qi lead to many different illnesses.

In fact, the importance of exercise shows up in many ancient medical texts. Hippocrates reportedly said, "Walking is man's best medicine." The famous 10th century physician Ibn Sina (Avicenna), too, wrote of the role of exercise in promoting health. Throughout history, there has been a consensus that exercise helps us maintain our physical and mental health.

Setting Up a Sustainable Exercise Program

So how much exercise is necessary? Currently, the American Heart Association recommends that people engage in 150 minutes a week of moderate activity or 75 minutes of moderate-to-vigorous activity. Ideally, people wouldn't go more than a day or two without exercising—

so exercising 30 minutes, 5 times a week, will provide more benefits than exercising for hours at a time, once a week. However, anything is better than nothing. If you've been sedentary and want to incorporate more exercise in your life, it may be better to start small and build up.

What Activities Are Best?

The most important question when you're deciding whether an activity belongs in your program isn't how many calories it burns or how healthy it is. It's whether you'll do it. Set yourself up for success by incorporating things you enjoy—or, at a minimum, activities you don't dislike—in your exercise routine.

If you've been inactive for a while, this can be difficult. Sometimes you need to think outside the box, to activities you haven't thought of as exercise. Do you like to dance, but you only do so at weddings? If so, now's a great time to check out a social dancing class through your local park district or community center. Maybe you find the idea of a treadmill boring, but you like bird watching or admiring architecture—if you do, think about adding in more nature hikes or walks through historic neighborhoods.

And don't be afraid to try something new. You might find that you enjoy the elliptical machine much more than the treadmill, or that you get a kick out of using a rowing machine. If you're competitive in other arenas, you might find that you can apply that competitive drive to games of tennis or racquetball.

Building in Variety

You've no doubt heard the apho-

STRESS AND BLOOD SUGAR

For people with diabetes, managing a stress response can be especially important. The stress hormones that cause the liver to secrete extra sugar into the blood in response to fear, anger, tension, or excitement also increase insulin resistance. For people without diabetes, the stress-induced rise in blood sugar is followed by an increase in insulin secretion, so the blood sugar spike is modest and momentary. For people with diabetes, however, stress can cause blood sugar to rise quickly and stay high for quite a while.

rism that variety is the spice of life. It's also the key to a sustainable exercise program. You want to build a program with different types of exercise activities. That way, you won't only exercise the same muscles and joints. Having several potential activities to choose from can also keep you from getting bored and cutting your exercise time short.

Think about the weather—don't rely on activities that can only be performed in good weather. Even if you get a gym membership, incorporate some activities that you can do at home, so that you're not reliant on a working car to exercise. If you travel a lot, look into things you can do on the road.

Different types of exercise will also provide different health benefits. Some activities improve cardiovascular health. Some examples of good aerobic activities include cycling, walking, running, dancing, rowing, and swimming. These are all activities that engage large muscles in repetitive movement and raise your heart rate and breathing for an extended period of time.

Cardiovascular, or aerobic, exercise will tone your muscles, strengthen your heart, improve blood flow throughout your body, and help improve your blood sugar levels. But it won't necessarily do much to make your muscles bigger (if you're a man) or denser (if you're a woman). Adding muscle requires strength training, such as weight lifting. And strength training has its own health benefits. It helps turn fat into muscle, and that improves your basal metabolic rate.

Your basal metabolic rate refers to the calories your body burns just to keep your heart beating, lungs breathing, eyes blinking...in other words, just to keep you alive. This calorie expenditure is like the interest you earn on a bank account: It's essentially something you get for doing nothing but being there.

Fat is metabolically stagnant. In other words, fat cells require virtually no calories to stay alive. Muscle, on the other hand, is very active metabolically. Muscle cells chew through a lot of calories even when they aren't moving. The more muscle you have, the higher your basal metabolism and the more calories your body burns all the time—even when you're resting.

Strength training involves moderate to high exertion for short periods of time. When a muscle is worked to near (but not quite) exhaustion, the muscle becomes stronger and more efficient. Stronger and more efficient muscles burn more calories every minute of the day, whether you are actively working them or not, and they can help you achieve your weight loss goals more quickly. Other types of exercise will improve flexibility and balance. There are especially important as we age.

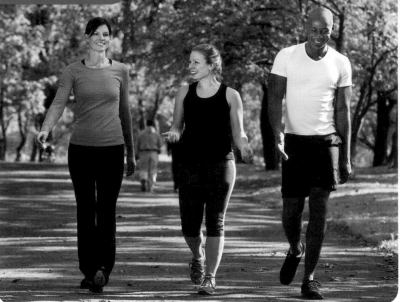

Walking for Health

Walking is so simple that we often overlook it as a form of exercise. But it has a lot of advantages. You don't need fancy gear or equipment. It's low impact. And you can fit a brisk 10-minute (or longer) walk into your way of life more easily than almost any other kind of exercise.

Although not as strenuous as jogging, walking will increase your heart rate and oxygen consumption enough to qualify as an aerobic exercise. When you walk, your heart starts to beat faster and move larger amounts of oxygen-rich blood around your body more forcefully. Your blood vessels expand to carry this oxygen. In your working muscles, unused blood vessels open up to permit a good pickup of oxygen and release of carbon dioxide. These changes improve your ability to process oxygen. And better circulation to your leg muscles can mean less leg fatigue and fewer aches.

The aerobic benefits aren't the only ones you'll get by incorporating walking into your life. Walking can refocus your attention from whatever is troubling you, reducing anxiety, tension, and stress. It helps you relax and recharge your mind and body.

Dealing with Aches and Pains

When some part of your body hurts, your first inclination may be to lie down and not move a muscle. While that can be appropriate when you first suffer an acute injury, it's precisely the wrong thing to do for other pain, such as chronic back pain, headaches, or arthritis. Remaining sedentary in those cases only makes matters worse.

Indeed, the more medical researchers learn about the body's response to pain,

the clearer it becomes that exercise is a key factor in pain management. What's more, exercise can often prevent the onset of pain in the first place by improving physical conditioning, which makes us less susceptible to the stresses, strains, and injuries that can result in pain.

No matter how carefully you exercise, you probably will experience a few little aches and pains—simply because you'll be asking your body to do things that it might not have done for years. Don't let a few minor physical discomforts discourage you. At the same time, don't persist in thinking that you should exercise until it hurts, or work through pain. Pay attention to your body.

Even people who have been exercising regularly complain of occasional soreness and stiffness. The pain may occur immediately following the activity or after some delay, usually 24 to 48 hours. Often the discomfort lasts for only a few days. It is practically impossible to completely avoid muscle soreness and stiffness. But you can reduce the intensity of the pain by planning your conditioning program so that you progress gradually, especially during the early stages. That approach will allow the muscles of the body to adapt themselves to the stress placed on them. If you become sore and stiff from physical activity, doing some additional light exercises or general activity will often provide temporary relief.

Muscle Cramps and Spasms

When one of your muscles contracts powerfully and painfully, you may have a muscle cramp. The contraction may occur at any time—at rest as well as during activity. Cramps usually occur without warning.

Among the causes of muscle cramps are fatigue; cold; imbalance of salt, potassium, and water levels; and overstretching of unconditioned muscles. You can reduce the chances of muscle cramps by maintaining a proper diet, making sure you warm up properly prior to vigorous activity, and stopping activity before you become extremely fatigued.

If a cramp does occur, it can usually be stopped by stretching the muscle affected and firmly kneading it. Applying

heat and massage to the area can restore circulation. If you're plagued with frequent cramps, drinking adequate fluid and eating foods with salt and potassium, along with muscle strengthening and stretching exercises, will usually eliminate the problem.

From the East

Many Westerners have been discovering the stress-reducing and pain-relieving benefits of exercise methods from across the ocean.

Qi gong and Tai Chi Chuan are centuries-old Chinese exercise forms. Adherents believe that qi gong stimulates and balances the qui, or life energy, flowing through the acupuncture meridians. Tai chi has been described as "meditation in motion." Its slow, gentle movements are reported to be helpful in releasing tension and relieving pain. For instance, Tai Chi-based exercises are approved by the Arthritis Foundation to help relieve pain.

YOGA

Yoga, from India, is another of the world's oldest health practices that has the

DO A SIMPLE QI GONG EXERCISE

The first step in performing a qi gong exercise is to locate the Dantian, a major energy center in the body near the solar plexus. The point is located below the naval at a distance equal to the width of four fingers. The acupuncture point located there is called "Gate to the Original Qi," and the Dantian is located inside the abdomen about a third of the distance between that point and the spine. This is the focus of meditation during qi gong exercises.

While performing qi gong, it's most important to relax and be calm. Sitting on the floor cross-legged or with legs extended, shoulders relaxed and hands facing down in your lap, meditate on the Dantian as you inhale normally. Continue focusing on your Dantian while you exhale normally, then slowly lean forward and slide your hands out in front of you on the floor. You should be fully stretched out by the end of the exhale, not forcing either the stretch or the breathing. Gradually sit up to the original position as you inhale, continuing your meditation on the energy center. Repeat for a few minutes, then discontinue the focused meditation and sit still with your eyes closed, breathing normally.

After a qi gong session, people typically feel energized and relaxed, ready to deal with the stresses of the world in a calm and grounded manner.

effects of elevating mood, reducing tension and fatigue, and putting people in a positive mood.

Most people have heard of yoga, but relatively few in the United States have ever practiced this ancient self-healing art. Although often associated with Eastern religions and practices, it is increasingly being adopted by Westerners for its numerous benefits. The most notable of these are increased circulation, better flexibility of muscles and joints, relaxation, and improved sleep.

Yoga is based on the principle that the mind, body, and spirit work in unison. If the body is sick, it affects the mind and spirit. If the mind is chronically restless and agitated, the health of the body and spirit will be affected. And if the spirit is depleted, the mind and body will suffer. There are many forms of yoga, many of which use various poses that incorporate stretching and breathing exercises to integrate mind, body, and spirit. (Don't worry: You don't have to lay on a bed of nails or twist your body into a pretzel shape to achieve yoga's benefits.)

Yoga can help by loosening tight muscles, releasing tension, and putting you into a deep state of relaxation. But it's a type of relaxation that requires fixed attention to work well. The breathing and stretching exercises are designed to slow down your racing thoughts and pull you into the present moment. The practice of yoga helps stem the flow of stress hormones that your body produces when you are under stress. Indeed, when your body, mind, and spirit are connected and relaxed, you are more resilient to stress. You will also undoubtedly sleep better.

Exercise #1

Lie on the floor or a bed with your arms near your sides and your legs slightly parted. Relax your entire body by letting it sink into the floor or bed. Breathe in slowly through your nose, and pull the air deeply into your lungs until you feel your abdomen rise. Slowly exhale. Be attentive to how your body feels as you breathe in and out. Repeat with as many breaths as you need to feel calm.

Exercise #2

Sitting comfortably in a straight-backed chair, with your back supported and legs uncrossed, practice the same breathing technique mentioned in the previous exercise. After two or three deep breaths, raise your hands above your head and stretch as if you were trying to touch the ceiling. Continue breathing while you stretch. Be attentive to how your body and your mind feel as you breathe. Repeat until you feel more relaxed and ready to sleep.

Exercise #3

Standing, with your feet shoulder-width apart, inhale deeply, clasp your hands together and raise them above your head, and gently raise up on your toes. Stretch your whole body upward. Exhale slowly as you bring your arms back down to your sides and lower your heels to the floor. Repeat one or two more times.

SELF-HYPNOSIS

Some people associate hypnosis with stage acts or television programs they've seen where people who were supposedly hypnotized acted like chickens or did other bizarre things simply because they were told to do them by the hypnotist. This stereotype conveys the impression that hypnosis is about losing control. But actually, it is about gaining control. A person who is truly hypnotized is in a deep state of relaxation and is fully aware of what is going on around them. For this very reason, self-hypnosis may prove helpful in relieving sleep problems associated with stress. It provides a tool that you can use to induce a deep state of relaxation whenever you want to.

There are many methods of self-hypnosis. Here's one that's fairly easy. Choose a positive statement that expresses a desire. For instance, "Each breath makes me feel more relaxed." Once you have the statement in mind, lie down and take three slow, deep breaths. Close your eyes and, starting at your head, begin using your affirmation statement on different parts of your body. "Each breath makes my forehead more relaxed." As you breathe, imagine releasing any tension in that part of your body when you exhale. Move to the next part: "Each breath makes my jaw more relaxed." Continue using the same affirmative statement with various parts of your body until you finish with your toes. Continue regular, slow, deep breaths throughout.

Then count backward from 100 to 95 and immediately imagine yourself being taken to a serene setting that you would like to visit. It could be indoors or outdoors, as long as it is peaceful and inviting to you. Once there, repeat your affirmation statement three times. Stay and enjoy the place for as long as you like. When you feel ready to leave, say goodbye to your special place. Then, before opening your eyes, tell yourself that you will slowly count from one to three and that by the time you reach three and open your eyes, you will feel fully relaxed.

GET SCREENED

If self-help techniques don't do the job, consider seeking professional help. Most mental health professionals are trained in helping clients deal effectively with stress. (A psychiatrist may also prescribe a temporary course of medication.) A mental health professional can also determine if clinical depression is playing a role.

EATING FOR BETTER HEALTH

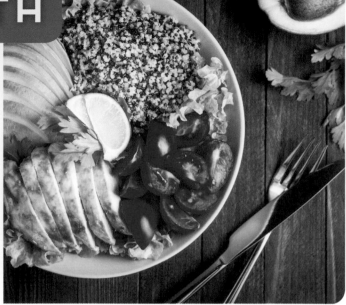

Many of the most common ailments we face today—from annoying problems like flatulence and constipation to more serious conditions such as heart disease and cancer—are linked to what we eat. Within the last several decades, the focus of research into possible links between nutrition and health has expanded; it now includes not only the potential dangers of eating certain foods (or too much of certain foods) but also the natural healing and protective powers that some foods possess.

That's not to say that food alone can cure disease or take the place of medical treatment. It is, however, becoming increasingly evident that food has disease-fighting potential. Translation? You have the power to choose foods that may help prevent and treat a host of today's most common maladies. If you follow nutrition news, you've probably heard how scientists have identified specific nutrients or substances that may play a role in preventing, causing, or treating certain diseases. But we eat foods, not just nutrients. And your overall diet is more than the sum of its parts. That's because substances in foods interact in powerful ways that can have profound effects on your health. So by trying to break your diet into artificial pieces and focus just on specific components, such as carbohydrates, protein, fat, vitamins, or minerals, you may end up overlooking some important foods and substances that have the potential to enhance your health and immune system.

In this chapter, you'll learn how to create an overall varied, balanced diet that promotes healing and good health. The major food groupings are presented in this section, with an emphasis on the specific foods and eating patterns that are known to provide health benefits. Here you'll find tips for choosing, storing, preparing, and serving various foods to preserve and enhance their disease-fighting potential. (You might be surprised to discover how much you can do to either protect or destroy a food's natural healing properties between the time you choose it at the store and the moment you put it in your mouth.)

When it comes to putting healing medicine in an easy-to-swallow package, Mother Nature has truly outdone science. Fortunately, science is catching on and gradually uncovering the many ways that food, especially food in its natural state, appears able to help the body heal and protect itself.

ANTIOXIDANTS

One term you'll hear a lot when it comes to food is that this food or that is "rich in antioxidants." So what does that mean? The antioxidant story begins with oxygen. We all know that oxygen is essential for life. Every cell in the body requires

oxygen to get energy from nutrients. Without it, our bodies would simply shut down. Ironically, though, the very same oxygen molecules that keep us alive are easily turned into rogue particles that can leave a path of destruction throughout the body. The damage they cause sets the stage for a variety of diseases and, scientists suspect, prompts many of the changes we associate with aging.

How can something so vital become so harmful? When an oxygen molecule is in its normal, beneficial form, the electrons in its chemical structure are paired off.

87

If that oxygen molecule loses one of its electrons, however, it becomes unstable—and destructive. This unstable molecule is called a free radical.

A free radical wants nothing more than to replace its missing electron, and it will steal one from wherever it can. If it robs a nearby oxygen molecule, that molecule becomes an unstable free radical. That destabilized molecule may, in turn, grab an electron from another molecule, causing a free-radical chain reaction. Alternately, an oxygen free radical may attack a nearby healthy cell, punching a hole in the cell's membrane to steal an electron and causing damage that may remain, even if the assaulted cell is able to replace its missing electron. The process in which oxygen free radicals assault stable molecules or healthy cells is called oxidation.

Free radicals can damage any tissue or organ, as well as any fat, protein, or carbohydrate molecule, in the body. The "victims" may include DNA, the genetic material that regulates cell growth; the fat molecules in every cell's protective membrane; the low-density lipoprotein (LDL) molecules that carry cholesterol in the bloodstream; and the proteins that help form the structure of the heart, blood vessels, muscles, skin, and other tissue. Down the road, these kinds of insults may accumulate and lead to inflammation, abnormal or uncontrolled cell growth, hardening of the arteries, and other disease-inducing changes. Among the diseases thought to be associated with free-radical damage are coronary heart disease, cancer, emphysema and other lung ailments, Parkinson's disease, rheumatoid arthritis and certain other immune-system disorders, cataracts and macular degeneration, and Alzheimer's disease and certain other dementias.

How does an oxygen molecule lose an electron in the first place? Sometimes, the loss occurs during the body's normal use of oxygen for metabolic processes. In other words, some free radicals are simply natural byproducts of living. But far more often, exposure to environmental toxins such as air pollution, cigarette smoke, and the sun's ultraviolet (UV) rays results in the creation of free radicals. Fortunately, our bodies have a natural defense mechanism against free-radical damage. The key element of that mechanism is a class of molecular compounds called antioxidants. Antioxidants neutralize free radicals, either by shielding healthy cells or by halting free-radical chain reactions. We have a number of antioxidant defenders at our disposal, each with its own protective functions. Some come in the form of vitamins and minerals. Vitamin C, vitamin E, and beta-carotene (a form of vitamin A) are antioxidants, as are the minerals selenium, manganese, and zinc. In addition, special chemicals from plants, called phytochemicals, can act as antioxidants in our bodies. We arm ourselves with these natural protective chemicals by eating a diet rich in plant foods, including vegetables, fruits, whole grains, legumes, and nuts.

Unfortunately, this antioxidant defense mechanism is not foolproof. It typically has little difficulty keeping up with the free radicals created by normal bodily functions, but it can be overwhelmed when we expose ourselves to too many environmental toxins and/or don't replenish our antioxidant stores by regularly consuming enough minimally processed plant foods (processing, as well as overcooking, tends to strip plant foods of some of their natural antioxidants). The resulting oxidative stress is thought to set the stage for the various diseases associated with free-radical damage. The good news is we can reduce our exposure to many environmental causes of free radicals. Plus, we can bolster our defenses against free-radical damage by boosting our dietary intake of antioxidants. In the rest of the chapter, we'll look at different kinds of foods and their different health benefits, including antioxidant properties.

FRUITS AND VEGETABLES

You've heard it before—and you'll hear it again. Eat your fruits and vegetables! There is no doubt that a diet with plenty of fruits and vegetables offers a whole host of health benefits, including protection from heart disease, stroke, high blood pressure, some types of cancer, eye disease, and gastrointestinal troubles. It can even help beat back the effects of aging. Some fruits and vegetables are good sources of vitamin A, while others are rich in vitamin C, folate, and potassium. Almost all are naturally low in fat and calories, none have cholesterol, and many are great sources of fiber. Fruits and vegetables also add wonderful flavors, textures, and colors to your diet.

Eat a Rainbow

If you haven't been eating much in the way of produce, choosing

any kind of fruit or vegetable more often is a great start. But to get the biggest bang for your bite, think in color. Choosing assorted colors of fruits and vegetables is a great strategy for making sure you get the most nutritional value from your produce choices. In many cases, the deeper and darker the color of the fruit or vegetable, the greater the amount of nutrients it contains. For example, spinach offers eight times more vitamin C than does iceberg lettuce, and a ruby red grapefruit offers 25 times more vitamin A than a white grapefruit. Yet every fruit and vegetable has a unique complement of vitamins, minerals, fiber, and phytonutrients that provide benefits. So it's important to sample from the complete color spectrum as well as to eat a variety within each color group. Here are some ideas to expand your produce palette.

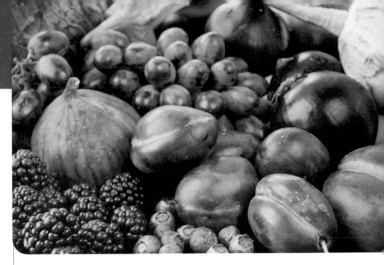

Blue/Purple

These fruits and vegetables contain varying amounts of health-promoting phytonutrients, such as polyphenols and anthocyanins. The pigments that give these foods their rich color pack a powerful antioxidant punch. Blue and purple produce give you extra protection against some types of cancer and urinary tract infections, plus they may help boost brain health and vision.

Fruits

- Blackberries
- Blueberries
- Currants, black
- Elderberries
- Figs, purple
- Grapes, purple
- Plums
- Prunes
- Raisins

Vegetables

- Asparagus, purple
- Belgian endive, purple
- Cabbage, purple
- Carrots, purple
- Eggplant
- Peppers, purple
- Potatoes, purple-fleshed

Green

Green fruits and vegetables contain varying amounts of potent phytochemicals, such as lutein and indoles, as well as other essential nutrients. These substances can help lower cancer risk, improve eye health, and keep bones and teeth strong.

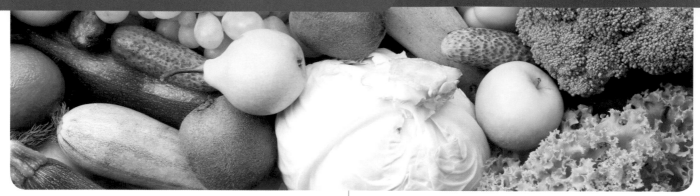

Fruits

- Apples, green
- Avocados
- Grapes, green
- Honeydew
- Kiwifruit
- Limes
- Pears, green

Vegetables

- Artichokes
- Arugula
- Asparagus
- Beans, green
- Broccoflower
- Broccoli
- Broccoli rabe
- Brussels sprouts
- Cabbage, Chinese
- Cabbage, green
- Celery
- Chayote squash
- Cucumbers
- Endive
- Greens, leafy
- Leeks
- Lettuce
- Onions, green
- Okra
- Peas, green (or English)
- Peas, snow
- Peas, sugar snap
- Peppers, green
- Spinach
- Watercress
- Zucchini

White/Tan/Brown

White, tan, and brown fruits and vegetables contain varying amounts of phytonutrients, such as allicin, found in the onion family. These fruits and vegetables play a role in heart health by helping you maintain healthy cholesterol levels, and they may lower the risk of some types of cancer.

Fruits

- Bananas
- Dates
- Nectarines, white
- Peaches, white
- Pears, brown
- Vegetables
- Cauliflower
- Corn, white
- Garlic
- Ginger
- Jerusalem artichoke
- Jicama
- Kohlrabi
- Mushrooms

- Onions
- Parsnips
- Potatoes, white-fleshed
- Shallots
- Turnips

Yellow/Orange

Orange and yellow fruits and vegetables contain varying amounts of antioxidants, such as vitamin C, as well as other phytonutrients, including carotenoids and bioflavonoids. These substances may help promote heart and vision health and a healthy immune system; they may also help to ward off cancer.

Fruits

- Apples, yellow
- Apricots
- Cantaloupe

- Cape gooseberries
- Figs, yellow
- Grapefruit
- Kiwifruit, golden
- Lemons
- Mangoes
- Nectarines
- Oranges
- Papaya
- Peaches
- Pears, yellow
- Persimmons
- Pineapple
- Tangerines
- Watermelon, yellow

Vegetables

- Beets, yellow
- Carrots
- Corn, sweet
- Peppers, yellow
- Potatoes, yellow
- Pumpkin
- Rutabagas

- Squash, butternut
- Squash, yellow summer
- Squash, yellow winter
- Sweet potatoes
- Tomatoes, yellow

Red

Phytonutrients in red produce that have health-promoting properties include lycopene, ellagic acid, and anthocyanins. Red fruits and vegetables may help maintain heart health, memory function, and urinary tract health and lower the risk of some types of cancer.

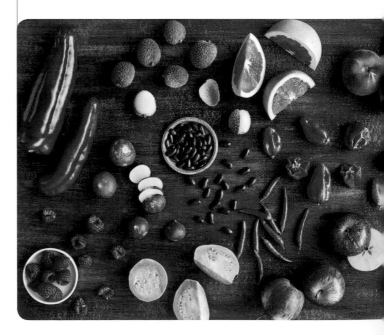

Fruits

- Apples, red
- Cherries
- Cranberries
- Grapefruit, pink/red
- Grapes, red
- Oranges, blood
- Pears, red
- Pomegranates
- Raspberries
- Strawberries
- Watermelon

Vegetables

- Beets
- Onions, red
- Peppers, red
- Potatoes, red
- Radicchio
- Radishes
- Rhubarb
- Tomatoes

Fresh and Beyond

There are lots of easy, nutritious, and affordable ways to enjoy fruits and vegetables all year long:

- Buy in season. Some types of fresh produce are great buys year-round, such as bananas, apples, broccoli, potatoes, carrots, cabbage, and spinach. Other items are more affordable—and better tasting—at certain times of the year. If your community offers a farmer's market, be sure to frequent it for extra-fresh produce.

- Go for convenience. Try prewashed and/or precut salad greens, baby carrots, and chopped fresh vegetables. The time savings can be huge, and the waste very little.

- Can it. Canned goods can be a low-cost, convenient way to enjoy your fruits and vegetables. Canned fruits and vegetables generally are comparable in vitamins and fiber to their fresh and frozen counterparts. Look for fruits packed in juice or water. Wash away extra sugar from canned fruits and extra salt from canned vegetables by rinsing them under cold water after opening.

- Hit the sales. Look for great deals offered by your local grocery store. Often, bargain prices on fruits and vegetables are used to draw in customers. Check the food ads before you shop. Since you're looking for variety, try the items that are on sale, even if some are new to you.

- Join the cold rush. Flash-freezing of fruits and vegetables keeps all the important nutrients locked in tight. Frozen produce is handy to keep in your freezer for whenever you may need it. Look for mixtures of vegetables to use in soups or stir-frys or to just steam or microwave and eat. Look for fruits frozen without added sugar.

Is It Ripe Yet?

When shopping for fresh fruits, you'll want to consider ripeness. As fruit ripens, the starch turns to sugar, which gives fruits their characteristic sweet taste. Some fruits continue to ripen after they're harvested, while others do not. Whether or not a fruit continues to ripen determines its storage and shelf life. For fruits that continue to ripen, it's a good idea to select them at stages of ripeness so they're not all ripe at the same time.

FRUITS THAT WILL CONTINUE TO RIPEN

- Apricots
- Avocados
- Bananas
- Cantaloupe
- Kiwi
- Nectarines
- Peaches
- Pears
- Plums
- Tomatoes

Fruits that require additional ripening should be stored at room temperature until they reach the desired ripeness. To hasten the ripening of some fruits, such as pears and peaches, put them in a loosely closed paper bag. They'll be ready to eat in a day or two. If fruits become overly ripe, instead of tossing them, try trimming any blemishes, then cooking and puréeing the fruit to make sauces for dressings or desserts. Fruits that do not ripen after harvesting should be stored in a cool area, such as the refrigerator, until you are ready to eat them.

KEEPING YOUR PRODUCE NUTRITIOUS

Fruits and vegetables are naturally nutritious. It's how you store, clean, and prepare them that will determine how nutritious they are when you eat them.

Storage

Fresh, properly stored produce will be the most nutritious. To keep produce fresh longer, store it unwashed and uncut. With the exception of a few items, such as onions, garlic, potatoes, and winter squash, fresh produce should be stored in the refrigerator. Most produce items are best stored loose in crisper drawers, which have a slightly higher humidity. If your refrigerator doesn't have a crisper drawer, use moisture-resistant wrap or bags to hold your produce. Fruits and vegetables that have already been cut and/or washed should be covered tightly to prevent vitamin loss and stored on refrigerator shelves.

Cleaning

Wash your produce in clean water. This important step should be done for all fruits and vegetables, even for produce

FRUITS TO BUY RIPE AND READY TO EAT

- Apples
- Cherries
- Grapefruit
- Grapes
- Lemons
- Limes
- Oranges
- Pineapple
- Strawberries
- Tangerines
- Watermelon

such as melons and oranges that have skin or rinds that you don't plan to eat. That's because surface dirt or bacteria can contaminate your produce when you cut or peel it. Plan to wash your produce just before you're ready to eat or cook it to reduce spoilage caused by excess moisture. The one exception is lettuce—it remains crisp when you wash and refrigerate it for later use. It is not advisable to use detergent when washing fruits and vegetables. Produce is porous and can absorb the detergent, which leaves a soapy residue. Special produce rinses or sprays can help loosen surface dirt and waxes.

Clean thicker-skinned vegetables and fruits with a soft-bristled brush. Peel and discard outer leaves or rinds. If you plan to eat the nutrient-rich skin of hearty vegetables, such as potatoes, and carrots, scrub the skin well with a soft-bristled brush. For cleaning fragile berries, such as strawberries, raspberries, blackberries, and blueberries, the best method is to spray them with the kitchen-sink sprayer. Use a colander so dirt and water can drain, and gently turn the fruit as you spray it.

Preparation

There are plenty of ways to enjoy your fruits and vegetables. Eat them raw whenever possible to get maximum nutrition. For vegetables that require cooking, such as asparagus, green beans, or Brussels sprouts, cook as quickly as possible—just until tender crisp.

MAXIMIZE THE FIBER

Did you know the fiber content of different forms of the same food can vary considerably?

- Raw apple with skin: 3.5 grams of fiber
- $\frac{1}{2}$ cup applesauce: 1.5 grams of fiber
- $\frac{3}{4}$ cup apple juice: little or no fiber

In the above example, the skin offers much of the fiber. Here's another example with a different slant.

- 1 cup raw spinach: about 1 gram of fiber
- 1 cup cooked spinach: about 3 grams of fiber

In this case, the spinach cooks down so you're eating a larger amount of the raw equivalent and thus getting more fiber.

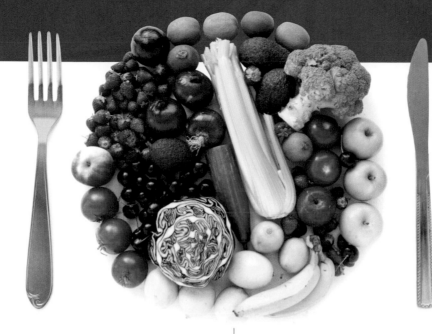

This helps to minimize loss of nutrients and also helps vegetables retain their bright color and flavor. Cook vegetables (and fruits) in a covered pot with just a little water—to help create steam that speeds cooking. Or try cooking in the microwave. This fast method of cooking helps to retain nutrients, flavor, and crispness.

Easy Ways to Get Your Helpings

- Start your day with fruit—add fresh or dried fruit to cereal, yogurt, pancakes, or waffles, or just enjoy it alone.

- Mix chopped vegetables into scrambled eggs, or fold them into an omelet.

- First, freeze fresh fruits, such as grapes, blueberries, and chunks of bananas, peaches, or mango. Then, enjoy them as a refreshing snack, or mix them with yogurt and juice in a blender to make a smoothie.

- Snack on a trail mix of crunchy, whole-grain cereal, dried fruits, and chopped, toasted almonds.

- Bring a prepackaged fruit cup, box of raisins, or piece of fruit with you to work or school for an energy-boosting snack.

- For a short-cut fruit salad, open two or more cans of chopped or sliced fruit and add some fresh or frozen fruits for a tasty and refreshing snack or meal accompaniment.

- Stuff a pita pocket with veggie chunks and sprouts, and drizzle on a low-fat ranch dressing.

- Toss pasta or rice with leftover vegetables, low-fat vinaigrette, and a sprinkling of shredded cheese or toasted pine nuts or almonds.

- Sneak in some extra helpings of produce by adding finely chopped vegetables, such as carrots, eggplant, broccoli, or cauliflower, to marinara sauce, soups, stews, and chili.

- Roast your vegetables for a deep, rich flavor. Drizzle them with a little olive oil, and roast in an oven set to 425 degrees Fahrenheit or on the grill until tender. Try carrots, asparagus, butternut squash, eggplant, broccoli—or just about any vegetable that strikes your fancy!

BREADS, CEREALS, RICE, AND PASTA

This group of foods has one thing in common—they are all made from grains. Any food made from wheat, rice, oats, corn, or another cereal is a grain product. Grain-based foods are rich in complex carbohydrates, your body's best energy source. As the body's key fuel, carbohydrates provide your brain, heart, and nervous system with a constant supply of energy to keep you moving, breathing, and thinking.

Grain products also supply B vitamins and iron (especially if they're enriched or include the whole grain), as well as other beneficial phytonutrients (substances in plants with health-protective effects). In addition, many grain-based foods supply fiber.

The "Whole" Story

An important strategy for choosing the best grain foods is to seek out products made from whole grains. A whole grain is the entire edible part of any grain, whether it's wheat, oats, corn, rice, or a more exotic grain. The three layers of a grain kernel each supply important nutrients:

- The outer protective coating, or bran, is packed with fiber, B vitamins, protein, and trace minerals.

- The endosperm supplies mostly carbohydrate and protein and some B vitamins.

- The germ is rich in B vitamins, vitamin E, trace minerals, antioxidants, and phytonutrients.

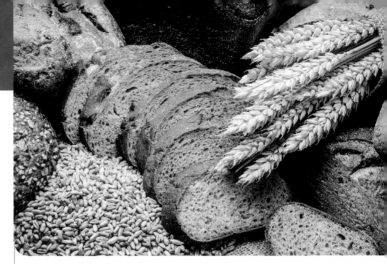

When whole grains are milled (refined), the bran and the germ portions are removed, leaving only the endosperm. Unfortunately, more than half the fiber and almost three-quarters of the vitamins and minerals are in the bran and germ. When you eat foods made from whole grains, you get the nutritional benefits of the entire grain. Enriched grain products add back some of the B vitamins—thiamin, folic acid, riboflavin, and niacin—and iron lost when the grain was milled. But lots of other nutrients and fiber don't get added back.

Whole-Grain Goodness

The individual nutrients in whole-grain foods—fiber, antioxidants, phytonutrients, and vitamins and minerals—each offer important health benefits of their own. When they work together in the "whole" food, however, they interact in powerful ways that help protect your health. For example, a diet rich in whole-grain foods is associated with lower risk for several chronic diseases and conditions including heart disease, cancer, diabetes, and gastrointestinal troubles. It can also play a role in the treatment of many of these diseases. A wide array of whole-grain foods is available in today's supermarkets.

Examples of foods that can be found in whole-grain versions include breads, ready-to-eat and hot cereals, brown rice, pasta, crackers, tortillas, pancakes, waffles, and muffins. You just need to know what to look for.

Get Your Whole Grain's Worth

When you're choosing among grain products, follow these tips to get the most fiber- and nutrient-filled forms.

Breakfast cereals:

- Look for "whole grain" on the front of the package.
- The words "whole grain" or "whole" appear in front of wheat, oats, rice, corn, barley, or another grain as the

first ingredient. Hint: Oats are always whole, even if they're rolled, instant, fine-cut, or coarse-cut.

- Breads, tortillas, and crackers:

- Look for "whole wheat" or "whole grain" in the product's name.

- A whole-grain flour, such as whole-wheat flour, should be the first ingredient listed. Wheat flour, enriched flour, and degerminated cornmeal are not whole grain.

Pasta and rice:

- Only brown rice is whole grain.

- Look for pasta made from whole-wheat flour. Hint: Some pastas are made with a mix of whole-wheat and white flours; they may be a good stepping stone or compromise if you're having trouble adjusting to the texture of whole-wheat-only pastas.

Your Daily Bread and More

Try some of these easy ways to make grains—especially whole grains— a regular part of your day.

- Get the first of your daily servings of whole grains from a whole-grain breakfast cereal.

- Use whole-wheat pasta in hearty soups, hot casseroles, and chilled salads.

- Make the switch to brown rice, or try a combination of brown and white rice.

- When you make bread, muffins, biscuits, cookies, pancakes, or waffles, substitute whole-wheat flour for half of the white flour, or add some oats, wheat germ, or bran cereal.

- Take a whole grain to lunch—a sandwich on whole-grain bread is one way to go, or add some new appeal to your lunchtime meal with a whole-grain bagel, roll, tortilla, or pita.

- Snack on popcorn, low-fat granola made with whole oats, brown-rice cakes, or snack mixes made with whole-grain cereal.

- Sprinkle wheat germ, oat bran, or bran cereal on yogurt, salads, or cut-up fruit. Or use it to coat fish or chicken or to top a tuna casserole. When you prepare a meat loaf or any meat mixture, add some bran cereal or wheat germ instead of bread crumbs.

- Be adventurous and try whole grains you've never tasted, such as whole-grain barley, bulgur, kasha, amaranth, quinoa, and couscous. Note: If you can't find whole-grain barley, choose scotch barley or pot barley, instead of pearled barley, which has lost a greater amount of fiber and nutrients in processing.

Grain Storage

All cereal should be stored in a dry location. Keep the inner bag folded down tightly to keep bugs out, or store the cereal in a container with a tight-fitting lid. Once opened, it'll keep for a few months before it goes stale, unless you live in a humid environment. If so, your best bet is to not buy the large box unless you know you'll finish it in a month or so. Another option is to transfer the cereal to a re-sealable plastic bag and refrigerate it.

Keep oats in a dark, dry location in a well-sealed container to keep bugs out. Store the container in the refrigerator if you live in a humid locale. The oats will keep up to a year. Whole oat groats are more likely to become rancid, so be sure to refrigerate them.

Dried pasta is fine stored in your cupboards for months, especially if transferred to airtight containers. Putting your colored pastas in see-through glass jars makes a pretty display, but they'll lose B vitamins that way; better to keep them cool and dry, away from light, and sealed up tight. Rice and other grains are also best stored in a cool, dark location.

Brown rice is more perishable than white rice. It keeps only about six months—slightly longer if you refrigerate it.

Because of its fat content, wheat germ goes rancid easily. Always store opened wheat germ in the refrigerator in a tightly sealed container. If you buy it in a jar, you can simply store it in the refrigerator in its original container. Fresh wheat germ should smell something like toasted nuts, not musty. Unopened, a sealed jar of wheat germ will keep for about one year. Once opened, it can keep up to nine months in the refrigerator if the jar is resealed tightly.

Whole-wheat breads may not have preservatives added. To prevent your bread from going stale, leave out at room temperature only as much as you'll eat in the next day or two, and keep it tightly closed in a plastic bag. Put the rest in the freezer. It defrosts quickly at room temperature if you take out one or two slices as needed. Or you can defrost a few slices in a jiffy in the microwave. But don't refrigerate your bread—it actually goes stale faster.

MEAT, POULTRY, FISH, BEANS, NUTS, AND SEEDS

Foods in this group are diverse, but they have something important in common—protein. The amount and quality of the protein in these foods vary, but all are considered high-protein foods. The animal foods contain high-quality, or complete, proteins, which means they supply all the amino acids your body needs to build the proteins used to support body functions. The plant sources of protein supply lesser amounts, and the proteins are not complete; all of the amino acids are not found in a single source, although plant sources can be combined to provide the amino acids needed to form complete proteins.

Besides protein, foods from this group supply varying amounts of other key nutrients, including iron, zinc, and B vitamins (thiamin, niacin, and vitamins B_6 and B_{12}). On the downside, some of the foods in this group contain higher amounts of fat and saturated fat. Some also include cholesterol.

Lean Red Meat

Could it be that red meat—wonderful, juicy, stick-to-your-ribs red meat—might actually have healing properties, other than the obvious way it makes your taste buds and tummy come alive? Why yes, yes it could. But you must honor the word "lean" in front. And you need to cast meat as a bit player rather than the main character in your meals (sorry, but that means no more eating an entire 16-ounce steak in one sitting). Lean red meat, including beef, veal, and pork (sometimes erroneously referred to as "the other white meat"), can indeed be part of a healthful diet. And they can contribute nutrients that may help you maintain good health and prevent or even fight disease.

Beef, veal, and pork are packed with high- quality protein. They are also the most nutrient-dense sources of iron and zinc, minerals that many Americans have trouble getting. While it is possible to get enough iron or zinc without eating meat, it's not easy. Eating lean meat is also a dandy way to get vitamin B_{12}, niacin, and vitamin B_6. So, including some lean meat in your diet can be nutritionally uplifting.

PUMPING IRON

The iron in red meat, especially beef, carries a double bonus. About half the iron in beef is heme iron, a highly usable form found only in animal products. And the absorption of the nonheme iron in meat is enhanced by the fact that it's in meat. Eating meat also enhances the absorption of non-heme iron from plant foods. (That's also a good reason to use smaller portions of meat mixed with plant foods in your meals.) The zinc in meat is absorbed better than the zinc in grains and legumes, as well.

Despite the bad press red meat has sometimes received, some research has shown that eating lean beef, veal, and pork is just as effective in lowering bad LDL cholesterol and raising good HDL cholesterol in your blood as eating lean poultry and fish is. Plus, close to

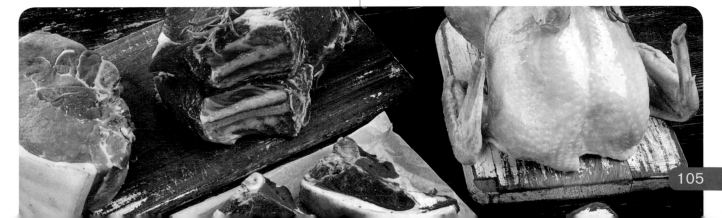

half the fat in lean beef is monounsaturated, the kind that helps lower blood cholesterol and reduce the risk of heart disease when it replaces saturated fat in the diet. And the saturated fat that beef does contain is stearic acid, a form that doesn't appear to raise blood cholesterol the way other saturated fats do.

Selection and Storage

The secrets to fitting red meat into a healthful eating plan are choosing lean cuts, trimming visible fat, preparing them without adding fat, and eating reasonable portions. When selecting red meat, here are some tips for finding the "skinniest" cuts.

Beef: Look for beef cuts with "loin" or "round" in the name, such as top round, round tip, top sirloin, bottom round, top loin, and tenderloin.

Veal: Lean cuts include cutlet, blade or arm steak, rib roast, and rib or loin chop.

Pork or lamb: Look for cuts with "loin" or "leg" in the name. Pork cuts include tenderloin, top loin roast, top loin chop, center loin chop, sirloin roast, and loin rib chop. Lamb cuts include leg, loin chop, arm chop, and foreshanks.

You can also look for cuts labeled "lean" or "extra lean." But don't be confused by ground beef labeled with a number followed by "percent lean." This refers to the weight of the lean meat versus the fat. For the leanest ground beef, simply look for ground beef that is at least 95 percent lean—it contains about five grams of total fat per three-ounce serving. Or look for ground round, which is the leanest, followed by ground sirloin, ground chuck, then regular ground beef.

When it comes to portions, forget the half-pound steak. To put a reasonable portion in perspective, three ounces of meat is about the size of your palm or a deck of playing cards. If you choose to eat all of your meat group servings at one meal, you can enjoy a steak that weighs about six to seven ounces or is about the size of two decks of cards. Or you can include a smaller portion of meat as a side dish and load up on vegetables and grains instead.

No matter the cut, choose meat that looks evenly red (grayish-pink for veal and pork) and not dried out. Refrigerate all meat as soon as you get it home. Place it on a plate so drippings won't contaminate other foods. If you don't plan to cook the meat within three to four days (one to two days for ground meat), freeze it.

Preparation and Serving Tips

Defrost meat in the refrigerator, in the microwave, or sitting in cold water that you change every hour. Never let it sit out at room temperature, which invites bacteria to multiply.

Choose your cooking method to match your cut of meat. Some lean cuts, such as beef cuts from the round, do better with a method that includes a liquid, such as braising or stewing. Grilling, roasting, broiling, and pan-frying work well for beef loin cuts. To minimize risk of foodborne illness, be sure ground meat is cooked until the internal temperature is 160 degrees Fahrenheit—or until the center is no longer pink and juices run clear. Roasts and steaks should be cooked until the internal temperature is at least 145 degrees Fahrenheit. Pork needs to cook to an internal temperature of at least 160 degrees Fahrenheit.

Trim all visible fat from meat before cooking. If you cannot buy ground meat as lean as you like, you can reduce the fat by placing cooked ground meat in a colander and pouring hot water over it. To tenderize tough lean cuts, try marinating, which also adds flavor, or do it the old-fashioned way and pound your meat with a mallet to break down the connective tissue.

Poultry

Chicken and turkey are often considered healthy, low-fat alternatives to beef, but that's not always true. A piece of dark meat, such as a chicken thigh with the skin on, can carry a hefty fat load. You have to make the right poultry choices to really save on fat. Your best bet? Skinless white-meat chicken or turkey. It's lowest in fat and calories.

ONE STEP FORWARD

Removing the skin before eating poultry saves fat and calories. But you quickly lose your low-fat advantage if you deep-fry it, smother it in fatty sauces or gravies, or cover it with cheese.

If you're trying to cut back on fat, skinless white-meat poultry offers a great low-fat protein option. You should be aware, however, that chicken and turkey contain about the same amount of cholesterol per serving as beef. Poultry is a generous source of some B vitamins that aren't as plentiful in beef, but it is only a fair source of iron.

Ground turkey is also available, but often it's higher in fat than you might think because it also contains ground turkey skin. For a truly low-fat ground turkey, look for "ground turkey breast."

RECONSIDERING THE EGG

Eggs were once considered too high in cholesterol and fat to have a place on a heart-healthy menu. Many people still hold to the outdated advice to limit eggs to one or two a week. But unless you're following a very low-fat diet and your doctor insists on it, you can probably safely increase your weekly egg allowance. It turns out that for most people dietary cholesterol has only a small effect in terms of raising blood cholesterol. Rather, it's saturated fat in the diet that has the greatest effect in causing blood cholesterol levels to rise. In studies where healthy participants ate up to one egg per day, there was no detectable effect on heart disease.

Selection and Storage

When choosing a whole chicken or turkey, look for one that is plump and firm with skin that looks moist and supple. The skin should have a creamy white or yellowish color (color varies depending on what the bird was fed), and it should have no odor.

Poultry is a highly perishable food that presents a standing invitation to bacteria if it's not stored properly. If you buy a fresh, whole chicken or turkey, be sure to store it right away in the coldest part of your refrigerator and use it within two to three days. If you don't plan to use it within that time, wash it, dry it, cut it into parts, wrap it, and freeze it. It will keep for up to nine months. If you freeze it whole, it will keep for one year.

Never let poultry thaw at room temperature. Thaw it in the refrigerator, and set it on a plate to catch drippings. It will take anywhere from one to two days to thaw a small 8- to 12-pound turkey, four to five days for a 20-pounder.

When you handle raw poultry, be sure to wash your hands thoroughly afterward with soap and warm water before you touch any other food or utensil. Also be sure to wash well the cutting board and utensils used during preparation. Skip this important food-safety step and you're risking cross contamination—transferring bacteria like salmonella from raw poultry to other foods served at the meal. Cooking kills salmonella bacteria, but if the bug is transferred to a raw salad, for example, an unpleasant case of food poisoning can result.

If you marinate chicken or turkey, do it in the refrigerator, not on the kitchen counter at room temperature. And don't use the marinade as a sauce for the cooked bird unless you boil the marinade before serving.

Though fried chicken is an American favorite, especially the fast-food variety, it's also loaded with fat. Opt for lower-fat methods of preparation. Roasting is a good fat-saving cooking technique for whole chickens and turkeys. Skinless chicken or turkey breasts are perfect for marinating in low-fat sauces or, when cut up and mixed with vegetables, for stir-frying. Chicken or turkey breasts also work well on the grill. If you want to add a sauce, wait until the poultry is almost done. Spread it on any sooner and it could scorch and burn before the breast is cooked all the way through.

No matter how you prepare chicken or turkey, be sure it's cooked thoroughly to an internal temperature of 180 degrees Fahrenheit for whole birds and dark meat and to 170 degrees Fahrenheit for boneless roasts and breast meat— the meat should be white, not pink, and the juices should run clear.

Standard advice has long been to remove the skin of chicken or turkey before you cook it to save fat and calories. But it turns out that fat and calories are about the same whether the skin is removed before or after cooking. Since skinless poultry tends to dry out during cooking, keep the skin on while cooking to hold in moisture and flavor. Just remember to remove the skin and any fat left behind before eating.

Fish

Fish makes a fabulous addition to any healthy diet. Its generally low fat content (many types provide 20 percent or less of calories from fat) makes it a great protein option. And the fat it does contain appears to hold promise in terms of preventing and healing disease.

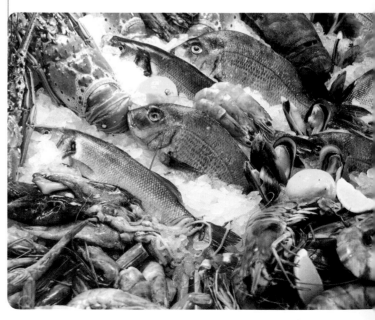

RISKY FISH?

In contrast to its potential healing properties, fish has been dogged by safety questions. Pesticides, mercury, and chemicals such as PCBs sometimes find their way into fish.

Fattier fish, which is richer in omega-3s, is also more likely to have greater amounts of environmental contaminants. Still, there are precautions you can take to reduce your risk of eating contaminated fish.

- Eat fish from a variety of sources.

- Opt for open-ocean fish and farmed fish over freshwater fish; they are less likely to harbor toxins.

- Eat smaller, younger fish. Older fish are more likely to have accumulated chemicals in their fatty tissues.

- Before you cast or drop your line, check the state's advisories for the waters you intend to fish to see if they advise limiting or avoiding consumption of fish from those waters.

- Avoid swordfish, shark, king mackerel, and tilefish, which are likely to be heavily contaminated with mercury.

Eating fish instead of meat or poultry usually means less total fat, but it almost always means less saturated fat (as long as you're not ordering a deep-fried fillet and smothering it with tartar sauce). And that's important when it comes to the health of your heart and blood vessels. Ironically, though, fatty fish are better for you than lean fish, because they contain more omega-3 fatty acids.

Two omega-3 fats, eicosapentaenoic acid (EPA) and docosahexaenoic acid (DHA), do a ton of good for your heart. EPA reduces the stickiness of blood platelets, preventing blood clots that can lead to heart attack and stroke. They also reduce triglyceride levels. DHA helps prevent irregular heartbeats by stabilizing electrical activity in the heart. One study has linked omega-3s with less risk of sudden cardiac death. Another found that older people who eat just one serving of fatty fish a week are 44 percent less likely to die from a heart attack. More research has confirmed the benefits of eating fish for both men and women. The Physician's Health Study of 22,000 men, for example, found that those with the highest blood levels of omega-3s had the least risk of sudden death. And the Nurses' Health Study of 85,000 women found two to four servings a week reduced heart-disease risk by one-third. Even those who ate fish as little as one to three times a month showed benefits. As a result of much of this research, the American Heart Association recommends two weekly servings of fish. (Supplements of fish oils, on the other hand, are not generally recommended by medical experts because higher doses—which are possible with supplements but improbable through consumption of fish—may cause problems with bleeding.)

Omega-3s have also shown promise in easing symptoms of rheumatoid arthritis because of their anti-inflammatory properties. Again, adding fish to the menu just two to three times a week has been suggested as a sound starting point.

You don't have to buy fresh to get the health benefits that omega-3 fatty acids offer. Canned fish, including tuna, sardines, and salmon, offer the same omega-3s as fresh varieties.

Selection and Storage

Fish doesn't stay fresh long. If handled properly, fatty fish, such as bluefish, tuna, salmon, mackerel, or herring, lasts only about a week after leaving the water; lean fish, such as cod, haddock, or perch, lasts about ten days. To be sure the fish you buy is fresh, check for a "fishy" smell. If you detect one, don't buy it. Whether you buy whole fish, fish fillets, or steaks, the fish should be firm, not soft, to the touch. The scales should be shiny and clean, not slimy. Check the eyes; they should be clear, not cloudy, and should be bulging, not sunken. Fish fillets and steaks should be moist; steer clear if they look dried or curled around the edges.

It's best to cook fresh fish the same day you buy it. (Fish generally spoils faster than beef or chicken, and whole fish generally keeps better than steaks or fillets.) But it will keep in the refrigerator overnight if you place it in a plastic bag over a bowl of ice. If you need to keep it longer, freeze it. The quality of the fish is better retained if the fish is frozen quickly, so it's best to freeze fish whole only if it weighs two pounds or less. Larger fish should be cut into pieces, steaks, or fillets. Lean fish will keep in the freezer for up to six months; fatty fish, only about three months.

Preparation and Serving Tips

Preparing fish without adding lots of fat is simple. The key to keeping fish moist and flavorful lies in taking advantage of fish's natural fat and juices. The number one rule: Preserve moistness. In practical terms, that means avoiding direct heat, especially when preparing lean fish.

You'll get the best results with lean fish, such as flounder, monkfish, pike, and red snapper, if you use moist-heat methods, including poaching, steaming, or baking with vegetables or a sauce that holds moisture in. Dry-heat methods, such as baking, broiling, and grilling, work well for fattier fish.

Marinades do wonders for fish.

> Fish cooks fast. That means that it can overcook quickly. You can tell fish is done when it looks opaque and the flesh just begins to flake with the touch of a fork. The general rule of thumb for cooking fish is to cook ten minutes per inch of thickness, measured at the fish's thickest point.

But as with poultry, keep safety in mind. Never marinate at room temperature; only in the refrigerator. And never use the marinade as a sauce for prepared fish unless you boil the marinade first.

Legumes (Dried Beans and Peas)

Legumes are a staple food all over the world. Dried beans and peas are one of the best sources of soluble fiber. Plus, they're low in fat and high in good quality protein—a great health-saving combination to appreciate.

Beans can be gassy, of course, but there are ways around that. So don't let their "explosive" nature scare you away from some of the best nutrition around. The soluble fiber in beans helps lower levels of damaging LDL cholesterol in the blood, thus lowering heart-disease risk. And by slowing down carbohydrate absorption, soluble bean fiber fends off unwanted peaks and valleys

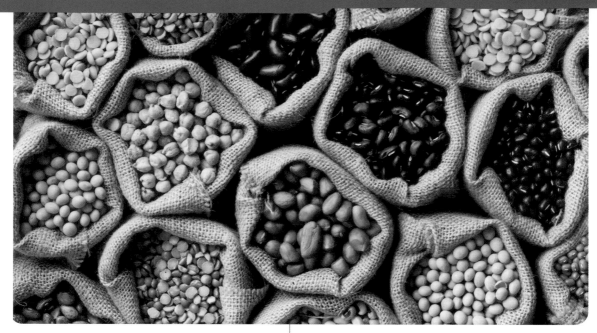

in blood glucose levels—especially valuable to people with diabetes.

Beans also provide substantial insoluble fiber, which can keep constipation and other digestive woes away. Legumes are also rich in folic acid, copper, iron, and magnesium—four nutrients many of us could use more of in our diets. In addition, dried beans and peas are generally good sources of iron, which is especially helpful for people who don't eat meat.

Selection and Storage

Dried beans are available year-round, are inexpensive, and can be found in any well-stocked grocery. You may need to visit a health-food store for more exotic varieties, such as Oriental azuki (or adzuki) beans, flageolets, cranberry beans, or yellow split peas.

If stored properly, dried beans and peas will last for a year or more. Keep them in their unopened bag. After opening, store the beans in a dry, tightly closed glass jar in a cool, dark spot. Note, too, that many varieties of beans are available already cooked and canned.

Preparation and Serving Tips

When cooking with dried varieties of

legumes, it's best to plan ahead. Before soaking or cooking, sort through the beans, discarding bad beans, pebbles, and debris. Then rinse the beans in cold water. It's best to soak your beans overnight, for six to eight hours; they'll cook faster and you'll get rid of gas-producing carbohydrates. But if you haven't planned far enough ahead, you can quick-soak for one hour. Quick-soak by putting the beans in water and boiling for one minute; then turn off the heat and let the beans stand in the same water for one hour. You may end up with a less-firm bean, however.

After soaking, discard any beans that float to the top, then throw out the soaking water and add fresh water to cook in. Add enough water to cover the beans plus two inches. Bring to a boil, then simmer, covered, until tender—about one to three hours, depending on the bean variety. They're done when you can easily stick them with a fork. Remember, cooked beans double or triple in volume.

Beans are notoriously bland-tasting, but that's what makes them versatile. They can take on the spices of any flavorful dish. Add them to soups, stews, salads, casseroles, and dips.

Nuts

This category is just a little nutty. It encompasses some foods that aren't true nuts but have been given honorary status due to their similar nutritional qualities. These include the peanut (really a legume), the Brazil nut, and the cashew (both technically seeds).

If you've relegated nuts to special occasions only, then it's time to reconsider. Because nuts are plant sources of fat, they are full of good-for-you monounsaturated and polyunsaturated fat, are cholesterol-free (unlike animal sources of fat), and are a good source of protein. Unsaturated fats are beneficial because they help keep your arteries healthy and help lower cholesterol levels. Some nuts (particularly walnuts) are also a good source of another type of heart-healthful unsaturated fat: omega-3 fatty acids. Studies are showing that omega-3 fatty acids can help lower cholesterol and blood-pressure levels, as well as reduce the risk of heart attack and stroke.

In one study, people who ate nuts—almonds, cashews, pistachios, walnuts, or peanuts—five or more times a week were half as likely to have a heart attack or suffer from heart disease as people who rarely or never ate nuts. This protective effect may be attributable to the healthy fat profile of nuts, or it may be the result of the vitamin E and fiber found in nuts, both of which can help stave off heart disease; perhaps it's these several attributes combined and even other as yet unidentified ones that played a role. Other studies have demonstrated that adults with a high blood cholesterol level can lower both their total and LDL cholesterol levels by substituting nuts for other snack foods.

CAUTION

Aflatoxin, a known carcinogen produced by a mold that grows naturally on peanuts, can be a problem. Discard peanuts that are discolored, shriveled, or moldy or that taste bad. And stick to commercial brands of peanut butter. A survey found that best-selling brands contained only trace amounts of aflatoxin, but supermarket brands had five times that much, and fresh-ground peanut butters—like those sold in health-food stores—averaged more than ten times as much as the best-selling brands.

Nuts are surprisingly good sources of vitamin E, which is considered an antioxidant nutrient. Antioxidants inhibit oxidation, a natural body process that causes cell damage, and have been linked to a lowered risk for several chronic diseases, including heart disease and some cancers. Nuts are also rich in potassium and magnesium, minerals that help the body function at its best by regulating blood pressure and keeping muscles and nerves working properly.

Nuts also offer a host of other nutrients, such as folate, phosphorus, copper, zinc, and selenium. Another bonus—nuts are so dense with nutrients that they quell hunger pangs with fewer calories compared to other snack foods that often provide calories with minimal nutrition.

Selection and Storage

Most fresh nuts are available only in the fall and winter. Shelled nuts can be purchased anytime. Look for a freshness date on the package or container. If you can, check to be sure there aren't a lot of shriveled or discolored nuts. Be wary if you buy your nuts in bulk; they should smell fresh, not rancid.

Because of their high fat content, you must protect nuts from rancidity. Nuts in their shells can be kept for a few months in a cool, dry location. But once they've been shelled or their containers opened, the best way to preserve them is to refrigerate or freeze them.

Preparation and Serving Tips

To munch on as a snack, nuts are pretty much a self-serve affair. For nuts that are tough to crack, use a nutcracker or even pliers. A nutpick is useful for walnuts. Brazil nuts open easier if you chill them first. Almonds can be peeled by boiling them, then dunking them in cold water. In cooking and baking, it's easy to get the nutritional benefits of nuts without overdosing on fat and calories, because a small amount of nuts adds a lot of flavor. Nuts sprinkled on your cereal can boost your morning fiber intake. Peanut butter makes a great snack on apple wedges or celery or simply spread on a piece of hearty whole-wheat toast. Walnuts go well tossed in Waldorf salad or with orange sections and spinach. Almonds dress up almost any vegetable when sprinkled on top. Nuts give grains extra pizzazz and crunch. Pignoli, or pine nuts, add a dash of Mediterranean flavor when included in pasta dishes; they're the nuts you'll find in your pesto dishes. Nuts stirred into yogurt make it a more satisfying light meal. And spice-cake and quick-bread mixes as well as pancake batters produce extra-special results when nuts are added in.

Seeds

Seeds are the "eggs" that contain the nutrients needed to nourish the growth of a new plant. So their high nutrient content shouldn't come as a surprise. What's surprising is that we generally relegate these nutritional wonders to the occasional snack rather than making them staples of our diet. With their gold mine of healthy minerals and their niacin and folic-acid contents, seeds are an excellent nutrition package. They are among the better plant sources of iron and zinc. In fact, one ounce of pumpkin seeds contains almost twice as much iron as three ounces of skinless chicken breast. And they provide more fiber per ounce than nuts. They are also good sources of protein.

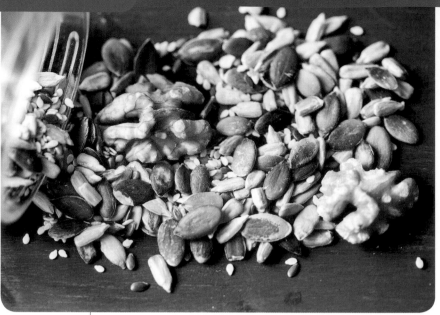

Sesame seeds are a surprising source of the bone-building mineral calcium, great news for folks who have trouble tolerating dairy products. And seeds are a rich source of vitamin E. The only drawback: Some seeds are quite high in fat. Sunflower and sesame seeds provide about 80 percent of their calories as fat, although the fat is mostly of the heart-smart unsaturated variety.

Selection and Storage

Seeds are often sold in bulk, either with their hulls (shells) in place or with their kernels separated out. Make sure the seeds you buy are fresh. Because of their high fat content, seeds are vulnerable to rancidity. If they're exposed to heat, light, or humidity, they're likely to become rancid much faster. A quick sniff of the seed bin should tell you if the contents are fresh or not. Seeds that still have their hulls intact should keep for several months if you store them in a cool, dry location. Seed kernels (seeds that have had their shells removed) will keep for a slightly shorter period of time.

Pumpkin and squash seeds are similar in appearance—both have a relatively thin hull that is white to yellowish in color. (Hulled pumpkin seeds are a popular ingredient in Mexican cooking.) Pumpkin-seed kernels are medium-dark green in color. Sunflower seeds are easily recognized with their hard black-and- white-striped hull.

Preparation and Serving Tips

You can't go overboard with seeds because of their high fat content. But, in moderation, seeds can be mixed with cereals or trail mix or eaten by themselves.

A sprinkling of seed kernels over fruits, vegetables, pastas, or salads adds a touch of crunchy texture and flavor. Sesame seeds are especially attractive as toppers for breads, rolls, salads, and even stir-fries.

MILK, YOGURT, AND CHEESE

Foods in this group supply approximately 75 percent of the calcium we consume. In addition, they provide protein, phosphorus, magnesium, and vitamins A, D, B_{12}, and riboflavin. Although milk, yogurt, and cheese offer significant amounts of calcium and other key nutrients, most people eat only half the recommended daily servings from this group. (And note that teens require more calcium than adults.) That means many people—adults and children—may not be getting enough calcium and other nutrients essential to staying healthy. Certainly, foods from other groups contain calcium, but foods outside this group generally contain less, and the body may not absorb it as well.

Also note: Other dairy-based foods, such as butter, cream cheese, and sour cream, are not considered dairy servings. These foods are made from the cream portion of milk and contain mostly fat and little, if any, calcium.

The Sunshine Vitamin

Vitamin D is an essential nutrient for building and maintaining strong bones and teeth. It is a unique vitamin—your body can make its own vitamin D when sunlight makes contact with your skin. To get enough, it only takes a few minutes of sun exposure, three times a week, on your hands, arms, or face (without sunscreen). However, if you live in Northern climates or don't get outdoors much, especially in the winter, you shouldn't rely on sunshine. Also, as you age, your body may not be as efficient at making vitamin D, so food sources become even more important.

Your most reliable source of vitamin D is milk. Although milk is fortified with the vitamin, dairy products made from milk such as cheese, yogurt, and ice cream are generally not fortified with vitamin D. Only a few foods, including fatty fish and fish oils, naturally contain significant amounts of vitamin D.

Other foods that contain smaller amounts of vitamin D include eggs, fortified breakfast cereals, and margarine.

CALCIUM FOR HEALTH

It is well known that calcium plays some pivotal roles in maintaining good health—from keeping bones healthy and strong and helping prevent high blood pressure to findings that the calcium in dairy products may make it easier to lose weight. Calcium also helps your blood to clot and keeps your muscles and nerves working properly. If your body doesn't get enough calcium from food, it steals calcium from your bones to help keep a steady amount in your blood.

Versatile Milk

There are many varieties of milk—with different flavors and nutrition profiles. The easiest way to enjoy milk is ice-cold with a meal or snack. Most types of milk have about the same amount of calcium, protein, and most other nutrients per cup. The main differences between them are in calories and fat.

Obviously, you're better off nutritionally if you choose skim, or at least 1 percent, milk to keep fat and excess calories to a minimum. However, if you have children under the age of two, give them whole milk. Young, rapidly growing children need the calories and fat that whole milk provides.

You might also want to give buttermilk a try. With its distinctively tart, sour taste, it's not for everyone, but many people prefer its flavor. Buttermilk is not as fattening as it sounds. Though originally a by-product of

butter, today buttermilk is made by adding bacteria cultures to fat-free or low-fat milk. Read the carton to be sure you're getting the low- or nonfat variety. Buttermilk tends to be saltier than regular milk, however (a concern if you have or are at risk for high blood pressure), and it may not be fortified with vitamins A and D.

Beyond Straight Up

There are other ways to include milk beyond drinking it plain:

- Many recipes call for milk, and in others, you can easily substitute milk for water. For example, use milk to make hot cereals; pancakes and waffles; soups; packaged potato, pasta, and rice mixes; baked goods; desserts; and drink mixes.

- Cereal and a cup of milk makes a good anytime snack—and it meets about a third of your daily requirement for calcium.

- Try blending milk with yogurt, fruit, and ice cubes for a

refreshing fruit smoothie. Add a flavor twist by using chocolate-, banana-, vanilla-, or strawberry-flavored milk.

- Have some coffee with your milk. Try a café latte or cappuccino to get a healthy amount of milk with your coffee.

- If you're a soda drinker, consider choosing fat-free milk instead of regular soda once in a while to save about 90 calories and get milk's nine essential nutrients.

Milk Storage

All milk should have a "sell by" date stamped on the carton. This date is the last day the milk should be sold if it is to remain fresh for home storage. It does not mean that you need to use it by that date. Generally, if milk is stored in a closed container at refrigerator temperatures, it will remain fresh for up to a week after the "sell by" date.

Pasteurization—the process of rapidly heating raw milk, holding it for a short specified period of time, then rapidly cooling it—removes most of the bacteria from milk. However, some of the remaining harmless bacteria can grow and multiply, although very slowly, at refrigerator temperatures, eventually causing the milk to spoil.

Store milk on a refrigerator shelf rather than in the door, which is not cold enough. To safeguard quality and freshness, store milk in the original container. Keep milk containers closed and away from strong-smelling foods. To avoid cross-contaminating milk, do not return unused milk from a serving pitcher to the original container. If milk has been left at room temperature for longer than two hours, throw it out.

PROTECT YOUR RIBOFLAVIN

Milk in plastic jugs is more susceptible to loss of riboflavin and vitamin A than milk in paperboard cartons. That's because light, even the fluorescent light in supermarkets, destroys these two light-sensitive nutrients.

You may find milk not only in the refrigerated section but also out on the shelf with packaged goods. This is called UHT (ultra-high-temperature) milk, referring to the processing technique. Though it must be refrigerated once you open it, unopened UHT milk will keep at room temperature for up to six months. UHT milk is just as nutritious as the milk you buy in the refrigerated section.

Drinking raw milk, or products that are made with raw milk such as some cheeses, can be risky. Raw milk has not been pasteurized and often carries bacteria that can make you sick. It's especially dangerous to give raw milk to children, the elderly, or people with impaired immune systems.

Cheese, Please

Cheese can be made from whole, low-fat, or skim milk or combinations of these. Regardless of the type of milk used to create it, cheese is a concentrated source of the nutrients naturally found in milk, including calcium. Indeed, many cheeses provide 200 to 300 milligrams of calcium per ounce.

"Low-fat cheese" used to be an oxymoron. No more. Today, there are dozens of reduced-fat, low-fat, and fat-free versions of American, cheddar, mozzarella, Swiss, and other cheeses, some you may find worth biting into. Fat in this new generation of cheeses has been cut anywhere from 25 to 100 percent. The average fat reduction is about 30 percent. Most of these contain added gums and stabilizers that help simulate the creamy texture and rich taste of full-fat cheeses.

The taste and texture of low-fat cheeses vary considerably. Some people find them fine substitutes for the full-fat

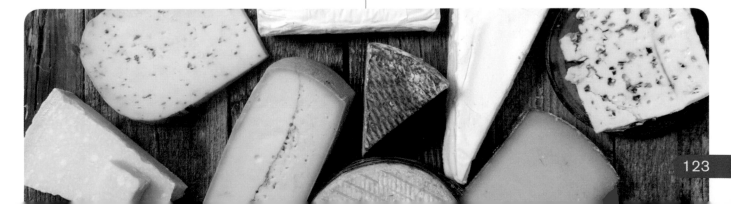

varieties, while other folks find they'd rather do without than settle for a low-fat substitute. Cheese connoisseurs will probably never be true fans of reduced-fat cheeses, but if you're trying to cut back on saturated fat and cholesterol, they do offer alternatives.

The one nutritional drawback of reduced-fat cheeses is that they are usually higher in sodium than full-fat natural cheeses. An ounce of regular Swiss cheese, for example, contains only about 74 milligrams of sodium. A reduced-fat Swiss may contain 300 to 400 milligrams or more per ounce.

Are reduced-fat cheeses the answer for a diet hopelessly high in fat? Hardly. Unless you're a big cheese eater, chances are other elements of your diet—such as fatty meats, whole milk, buttery muffins and croissants, chips, and ice cream—are more in need of a good fat-trimming. But substituting reduced-fat for full-fat cheese can't hurt. When it comes to the war on fat, every gram counts. Another option for cheese lovers is to use strong-flavored cheeses, such as Parmesan, blue, or gorgonzola. With these, a little

can go a long way in terms of adding flavor to dishes.

Selection and Storage

Many cheeses have considerably more fat per serving than a cup of milk. For reduced-fat cheeses, opt for varieties that provide no more than five grams of fat per ounce. Regular cheeses provide eight to nine grams per ounce.

Brands vary a lot in taste and texture. Shop around until you find one you like. You're better off choosing a reduced-fat cheese based on taste and then trying it in recipes.

Remember, the less fat a cheese contains, the harder it is to use in cooking. Because of their high moisture content, lower-fat cheeses turn moldy more quickly than their full-fat counterparts. Keep them well wrapped in the refrigerator and use them as soon as possible.

Cooking with Cheese

In general, the further you get from traditional cheese, in terms of fat content, the more careful you have to be about applying heat. It's the high fat content of regular cheese, generally about 70 percent of its calories, that gives full-fat cheese its smooth, creamy texture and allows it to melt easily. When you reduce the fat content, the cheese becomes less pliable and more difficult to melt.

The lower the fat content, the tougher the melting problem becomes. Trying to make a cheese sauce with a reduced-fat cheese can truly be an exercise in futility because the product is prone to breaking down into a clumpy, stringy mess.

Nonfat cheeses are best served "as is" in unheated sandwiches or in salads. They generally have milder flavors than regular cheeses and sometimes have what cheese purists sometimes describe as slightly "off" flavors.

To lighten the calorie and fat load of recipes without dramatically altering the flavor or texture, try replacing one-half to two-thirds of a full-fat cheese with a reduced-fat variety. Grated cheese blends best. Or combine a small amount of

full-fat, full-bodied cheese like extra sharp cheddar or Parmesan with a reduced-fat cheese. A little full-fat cheese can go a long way toward improving the flavor of the dish. Most reduced-fat cheeses melt smoothly when they are layered in a casserole; the layers serve as insulation and help prevent the cheese from separating or becoming stringy.

The lower the amount of fat in a cheese, the longer it takes to melt and the more likely it is to produce a "skin" and scorch when baked. To counter this problem, top casseroles and baked pasta dishes with reduced-fat cheese only near the end of the baking time, and heat until just melted. Serve immediately.

Meltability on top of dishes like casseroles or pizzas varies among varieties of reduced-fat cheeses just as it does among traditional cheeses. You may, for example, find a fat-reduced mozzarella melts much more smoothly than a fat-reduced cheddar. Meltability, texture, and taste may also vary among brands within a variety. Therefore, you'll probably need to do some shopping around and some experimenting to determine which of the varieties and which brands suit your needs and tastes in various situations; you'll probably prefer some kinds for snacking and other kinds for cooking or as toppings.

Say "Yes" to Yogurt

Yogurt was a long-established staple in Eastern Europe and the Middle East before it reached our shores. And there was a time when yogurt eaters in this country were considered "health nuts." Our attitudes have changed considerably. Today, yogurt is commonly consumed by men, women, and children of all ages. Walk into any supermarket today, and you'll see the varieties and flavors of this nutritious food take up considerable space in the dairy section.

Friendly Bacteria

Yogurt may not be the miracle food some have claimed, but it certainly has a lot to offer in the health department. Besides being an excellent source of bone-building calcium, it is believed that the bacterial cultures, Lactobacillus bulgaricus (*L. bulgaricus*) and Streptococcus thermophilus (*S. thermophilus*), that

are used to make yogurt carry their own health benefits. For example, research has suggested that eating yogurt regularly helps boost the body's immune-system function, warding off colds and possibly even helping to fend off cancer. It is also thought the friendly bacteria found in many types of yogurt can help prevent and even remedy diarrhea.

For people who suffer from lactose intolerance, yogurt is often well tolerated because live yogurt cultures produce lactase, making the lactose sugar in the yogurt easier to digest. But don't look to frozen yogurt as an option; most frozen yogurt contains little of the healthful bacteria.

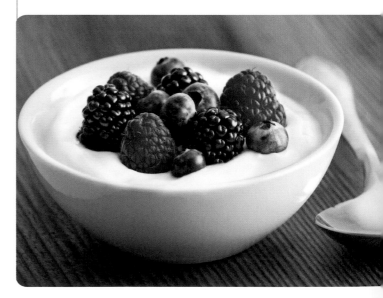

Yogurt Selection and Storage

There is a dizzying array of brands and flavors and varieties of yogurts in most supermarkets. But there are some basic traits to look for when deciding which to put in your grocery cart. Consider choosing plain, vanilla, lemon, or any one of the yogurts without a jamlike fruit mixture added. The mixture adds mainly calories and little if anything in the way of vitamins, minerals, or fiber. Your best health bet is to add your own fresh fruit to plain fat-free yogurt.

Yogurt must always be refrigerated. Each carton should have a "sell by" date stamped on it. It should be eaten within the week following the "sell by" date to take full advantage of the live and active cultures in the yogurt. As yogurt is stored, the amount of live and active cultures begins to decline.

Preparation and Serving Tips

Yogurt can be enjoyed as a low-fat dessert, snack, or meal accompaniment; just add sliced berries, nuts, wheat germ, bananas, peaches, fruit cocktail, mandarin-orange slices, pineapple chunks, low-fat granola, or bran cereal. Yogurt also works well as a low-fat substitute in a lot of recipes that call for high-fat ingredients such as sour cream or cream. Yogurt is especially well-suited as a base for vegetable and/or chip dips and salad dressings.

WHAT ABOUT CHOCOLATE?

It's the very definition of good news: Chocolate may be good for you! For years, chocolate has been looked upon as a decadent delight, craved for its lusciousness but banished to the "bad for you" food category. To the surprise of many health experts and the delight of chocolate-lovers everywhere, however, research has begun to reveal the healing potential hidden in the cacao beans from which chocolate is made. While these findings don't exactly elevate chocolate to the status of "health food," they do suggest that when it's chosen and enjoyed wisely, chocolate can have a place in a healing diet.

These properties don't negate chocolate's status as a high-calorie food, of course—especially the varieties most commonly consumed in the United

States. And it's unlikely the latest research will prompt nutritionists and doctors to recommend that we add lots of chocolate to our diets. But the promising evidence of healing potential does suggest chocolate may no longer need to be forbidden fruit. Making room in the diet for limited amounts of cacao-rich chocolate and cocoa may thrill our taste buds, quench our cravings, and play a role in good health.

Many of chocolate's health-promoting properties appear to stem from the antioxidants found in cacao beans.

Flavonoids: Cacao's Antioxidant Superstars

Researchers have discovered that cacao is rich in antioxidant phytochemicals, especially a type called polyphenols. Polyphenols are found not only in chocolate products but in fruits and fruit juices, vegetables, tea, coffee, red wine, and some grains and legumes. And the available research seems to strongly point to some role for polyphenols in preventing a variety of diseases.

The largest and most important class of polyphenols are the flavonoids. More than 5,000 flavonoids have been identified so far, and they have begun to attract a lot of attention for their potential health benefits. Among the flavonoid-rich foods that have shown promise lately are strawberries and blueberries, garlic, red wine, and tea. But these plant foods can't hold a candle to cacao-rich dark chocolate and cocoa products when it comes to flavonoid content and antioxidant power. Cocoa, for example, has almost twice the antioxidants found in red wine and close to three times the antioxidants in green tea, when compared in equal amounts.

One of the flavonoids in cacao (known as cocoa flavonoids, or cocoa polyphenols) gaining a particular reputation for healing is epicatechin. One Harvard Medical School scientist was so impressed by epicatechin's effects that he has said it should be considered essential for human health and, therefore, raised to the status of a vitamin. He's also stated that the health benefits of epicatechin are so striking that it may rival penicillin and anesthesia in terms of importance to public health. The researcher developed his views on epicatechin after spending years studying the health benefits of heavy cocoa drinking on an isolated tribe of people called the Kuna, who live on islands off the coast of Panama. The Kuna drink up to 40 cups of natural (unsweetened) cocoa per person every week. The Harvard scientist, working with an international team of colleagues, found that the island Kuna have remarkably low rates (less than 10 percent) of four of the five most common killer diseases in the industrialized world: heart disease, stroke, cancer, and diabetes. The research further indicates that the Kuna's high intake of epicatechin from their cocoa is a primary cause of the low disease rates. Indeed, when tribe members leave their isolated islands to settle on mainland Panama—where they drink far less of the natural cocoa—their disease rates rise.

In addition to demonstrating the healing potential of cocoa, the Kuna research highlights an important point about that potential. The Kuna not only drink large quantities of cocoa, the cocoa they drink has a very high flavonoid content—far higher than the flavonoid content of many of the sweetened, high-calorie, high-fat cocoa and chocolate products found on grocery-store shelves. And that's essential to its apparent health benefits. The Kuna grow their own cacao beans, gently roast and minimally process them, and use them to make an unadulterated cocoa that has a very high percentage of cocoa solids. And it's the cocoa solids that contain the flavonoids.

Flavonoids, however, also give natural chocolate a very bitter taste. So in an effort to please their sweet-toothed consumers, chocolate manufacturers have traditionally tried to tame that natural bitterness by removing flavonoids and/or masking their taste. Nearly every step of the typical processes that turn cacao beans into chocolate and cocoa, which include fermenting, roasting, and Dutching, removes some of the flavonoids. Likewise, adding ingredients such as sugar and milk to chocolate or cocoa—again, to mask or replace bitterness—leaves less room for cocoa solids and therefore results in a lower-flavonoid product.

While the rest of us cannot control the way our cacao beans are grown and processed, as the Kuna do, we can increase our chances of getting and benefiting from cocoa flavonoids by opting for cocoa and chocolates with the most cocoa solids and the least sugar and milk added.

In the past several years, scientists have produced some compelling research suggesting that cocoa flavonoids can help lower blood pressure, improve blood-vessel function, make blood less likely to form dangerous clots, and prevent the creation of artery-clogging blood-cholesterol molecules. All of these effects help ensure smooth, adequate, and uninterrupted blood flow to the heart and brain, lowering the risk of heart attack and stroke.

Chocolate is also a good source of certain vitamins and minerals your body needs to stay healthy, including vitamins C, D, and E; B-complex vitamins; and the minerals iron, copper, phosphorus, zinc, calcium, and potassium. Cocoa is also the greatest natural source of magnesium, a deficiency of which is associated with high blood pressure, heart disease, diabetes, joint problems, and premenstrual syndrome.

Selection and Usage

According to the government's Agricultural Research Service, when it comes to the common chocolate products that pack the most flavonoids and the greatest antioxidant punch, natural (rather than Dutched), unsweetened cocoa powders top the list. They also tend to be the lowest in calories and so can be the most weight-wise way to quench your chocolate desires. The process of Dutching, or alkalinizing, cocoa powder removes some of the natural flavonoids, so if you can find it, choose an un-Dutched dark-chocolate cocoa powder (not a milk-chocolate cocoa mix), and prepare it with water.

Sugar-sweetened powders retain fewer flavonoids—the sugar leaves less room for flavonoid-containing cocoa solids—and, of course, are higher in calories, so try an unsweetened powder (if you can't handle it unsweetened, you'll at least be able to add only as much sugar as is absolutely necessary) or, if you can find one, an artificially sweetened one.

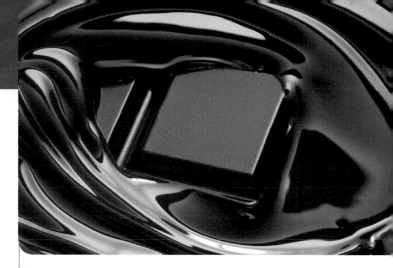

When it comes to solid chocolates, opt for dark chocolates. Milk chocolates typically have no more than half the amount of cocoa solids that dark chocolates contain—and therefore they have far fewer healing flavonoids and much less antioxidant power. With the added milk and sugar, milk chocolate bars simply have far less room for cocoa solids and are often considerably higher in empty calories (calories that provide no nutritional benefit other than energy). A typical milk chocolate bar contains 30 percent cacao, 20 percent milk solids, 1 percent vanilla and emulsifier, and 49 percent sugar. Some research even suggests that milk may interfere with the absorption of the antioxidants in cacao. And don't even bother with white chocolate if you're looking for any health benefits. It contains only cocoa butter, not cocoa solids (so no healing flavonoids), and loads of sugar.

How much chocolate and/or cocoa is it okay to consume? Moderation is absolutely key. If natural cocoa, especially an unsweetened variety, satisfies your taste for chocolate, that's definitely the way to go. You can probably enjoy a few cups a day. Because of its calorie content, however, you shouldn't look to add solid chocolate regularly to your diet unless you really enjoy it. That means that if you'd like to enjoy a square or two (but not much more) of cacao-rich dark chocolate every day, you'll need to cut back—by an equivalent number of calories or more—on other sugary or fatty foods you eat that day. Do not replace nutrient-rich foods, such as vegetables, fruit, and whole grains, with chocolate.

TEA

Tea has long been considered a healthful drink, and even thousands of years ago it was prescribed for a wide variety of ailments. Now research is revealing the science behind the ancient wisdom. Tea has healing properties that can help prevent diseases as dissimilar as heart disease and cancer.

Before tea became a beloved and much sought-after beverage worldwide, it was used medicinally. The Chinese credited it as a remedy for everything from headaches to melancholy. In recent years we've come full circle, and tea is once again being touted for its healing properties. Today we know what the ancient world did not: Tea has three active ingredients that contribute to its healing power—flavonoids, fluoride, and caffeine. But the flavonoids are responsible for most of tea's health benefits.

Go Green—with Flavonoids

Research has shown an indisputable link between eating plant foods and good health. Vegetables and fruits contain an array of vitamins, minerals, and phytochemicals, plant compounds that have health-protective and disease-preventive properties. Tea, which comes from the *Camellia sinensis* plant, also has an abundance of phytochemicals.

There are an estimated 3,000 varieties of tea produced worldwide. With so many different types of tea, you might think there are many different plants that produce them. But that's not the case: All tea leaves trace their roots to one plant. It's the processing the leaves undergo after they are harvested that determines whether they will become black, oolong (wu-long), green, or white tea. All true tea comes from the leaves of an evergreen shrub, *Camellia sinensis.*

Herbal tea is not really tea because it doesn't come from the *Camellia sinensis* plant. Herbal teas are tisanes, or infusions, of herb leaves, roots, seeds, or flowers in hot water. Some true teas, like Earl Grey, are black teas blended with an herb or essential oil. But unless a product contains leaves from the *Camellia sinensis* plant, it is not truly tea.

There are thousands of phytochemicals in plants. Tea leaves contain a subgroup called polyphenols, or tea polyphenols, that include flavonoids. Polyphenols—including flavonoids—are powerful antioxidants, which are critical to your health because they act as a kind of defense system for your body. In addition to their antioxidant activity, flavonoids can also help regulate how cells function. Tea is particularly high in flavonoids, higher than many vegetables or fruits. Tea provides about 83 percent of the total intake of flavonoids in the American adult diet, followed by citrus fruit juices (4 percent), and wine (2 percent), according to a 2007 study in the *American Journal of Nutrition.*

Among the foods and beverages tested, black tea provides the largest number of flavonols—a type of flavonoid—in the U.S. diet (32 percent), according to scientists in the Nutrient Data Laboratory at the USDA Agricultural Research Service.

Flavonoid Levels in Tea—The Ups and Downs

There are thousands of flavonoids, but one type called *catechins* is currently in the limelight. Of special interest is *epigallocatechin gallate* (EGCG), a compound that is thought to be an especially powerful antioxidant. Researchers believe EGCG may be a key to the development of new drugs or complementary therapies to treat disease. Other tea catechins called *epicatechin* (EC), *epigallocatechin* (EGC), and *epicatechin gallate* (ECG) are also being investigated.

Green and white tea have an abundance of EGCG—more than black or oolong, both of which contain many other types of antioxidants that scientists have studied for their healing benefits. In fact, a cup of green tea has more catechins than an apple.

Different kinds of tea have different kinds of flavonoids. That's important because different flavonoids appear to play different roles in protecting the body from disease. While green tea has the most EGCG, black and oolong teas have more of the complex flavonoids called thearubigins and teaflavins. These are formed during the fermentation process and have been found to offer protection against heart attacks and cardiovascular disease. Black, green, and oolong teas are a good source of the flavonols kaempferol, quercetin, and myricetin, which help relax blood vessels, improve blood flow, and reduce inflammation in cells, among other benefits.

Fluoride

The tea plant absorbs fluoride from the soil and from fertilizers, and the mineral accumulates in the leaves over time. The amount of fluoride in brewed tea varies depending on the type of leaf, the brewing time, and the amount of fluoride in the water. In general, higher quality tea, which is made from younger leaves, contains less fluoride.

That means white tea, which is made from the very youngest, unopened leaf buds, is unlikely to have much fluoride at all. Of the more common teas, oolong tea has the least fluoride (0.1–0.2 mg per 8 ounces) while black tea has the most (0.2–0.5 mg per 8 ounces). Green tea is in between the two with 0.3–0.4 mg per 8 ounces. Brick tea, a lower grade of tea made from older leaves and stems, has the most fluoride of all (0.5–1.7 mg per 8 ounces), but it is rarely consumed in the United States. The fluoride content provided above does not include the water in which the tea is brewed. In adequate doses, fluoride strengthens both teeth and bones, protecting against cavities and bone-density loss.

The U.S. Institute of Medicine recommends that adults get 3 to 4 mg of fluoride per day, and that children get 0.7 to 2 mg per day, depending on their age and body weight. A Japanese study found that rinsing the mouth

DAILY DOSE

Studies of green tea have tested the effects of drinking between 1 and 10 cups per day (containing 8 ounces each), with most studies using 4 cups per day as a possible therapeutic dose. This amounts to about 750 milligrams (mg) of EGCG, the most powerful antioxidant found in green tea. Brewed green tea has 188 mg of EGCG per cup, while black tea has 22 mg. You can buy green tea as an extract in pill form, but these products are not standardized, so they vary in strength. Currently there is no recommended daily dose.

with green tea prevented the production of acid as well as the growth of bacteria that cause cavities. And a small study in Italy found that drinking black tea helped prevent cavities and plaque. Too much fluoride, however, can cause fluorosis, a condition in which the teeth become mottled and discolored. In severe cases, the tooth enamel becomes soft and crumbly. Excess fluoride intake can also cause brittle bones.

Caffeine

Caffeine is a stimulant that increases heart rate, makes you alert, and revs up metabolism. All *Camellia sinensis* teas naturally contain caffeine, but the amount varies depending on the grade and type of tea, whether it is brewed from loose leaves or a tea bag, and how long it is brewed.

Black tea has the most caffeine (42 to 72 mg per 8 ounces) while green, white, and oolong teas have less (9 to 50 mg per 8 ounces). Compare those amounts with the caffeine content of coffee, which has 110 to 140 mg per 8 ounces. Decaffeinated teas only have 1 to 4 mg per 8 ounces.

TIME AND TEMPERATURE

One 2006 study in Taiwan found that the hotter the water, the faster the tea leaves would release antioxidants and caffeine into the brew. Steeping in cold water takes longer to produce a brew with the same level of antioxidants and caffeine.

Being Careful with Caffeine

While caffeine provides health benefits, it can cause problems when it interacts with certain medications. Caffeine is known to both enhance and interfere with certain drugs. For example, taking the antibiotic ciprofloxacin (*Cipro*) with caffeine can increase nervousness, anxiety, and heart pounding. Caffeine may interact with epinephrine, a drug used to treat severe allergic reactions and acute asthma attacks that don't respond to other asthma medication, causing dangerously high blood pressure. Because caffeine is a diuretic, it will increase the effects of diuretic drugs, which are often prescribed for high blood pressure.

And caffeine may interfere with the action of antianxiety or muscle-relaxant medications such as Valium and Ativan, and other psychoactive drugs, especially MAO inhibitors. Caffeine can increase the stomach's production of acid and can exacerbate the symptoms of acid reflux or ulcers.

Tea and Your Ticker

Heart disease is the leading cause of death in the United States, but tea drinking may be able to shrink that number. Some research shows that black and green tea both help fight the development of cardiovascular diseases including heart attack and stroke. A number of studies have shown that tea consumption can slow down the progression of atherosclerosis, or hardening of the arteries. Tea has also been shown to lower LDL, or "bad," cholesterol and relax blood vessels, which can lower blood pressure. These are all important steps in preventing heart disease. A 2002 University of North Carolina statistical review of many different tea studies found that people who drink three or more cups of black tea each day have a moderately reduced risk (about 11 percent) of heart disease and stroke compared to those who do not drink tea. The results of a Saudi national study, published in 2003, show a significantly lower incidence of heart disease among those who drank more than six cups of black tea per day compared to those who did not, even after adjusting for other risk factors such as smoking and age. The study compared tea consumption and the incidence of coronary heart disease in 3,430 Saudi Arabian men and women between the ages of 30 and 70. Those who drank black tea were found to have lower cholesterol and triglyceride levels as well.

Green tea seems to offer cardiovascular protection, too. An 11-year study that followed the tea consumption of more than 40,000 people in Japan found that people who drank more than five cups of green tea a day were 26 percent less likely to die of cardiovascular disease during the study period and 16 percent less likely to die from any cause at all. Another large study of overall diet in Japan published in 2007 found that people who drank green tea in addition to eating a traditional Japanese diet of fruits, vegetables, soy, and seaweed had a significantly lower incidence of cardiovascular disease than those whose diets were higher in red meat and dairy and lower in tea. This was evident despite the healthier group's tendency to consume more sodium and to have high blood pressure.

Cancer

All kinds of tea have been studied for their effects against various cancers, both in laboratory and human studies, with mixed results. Scientists caution that it's too soon to tell for sure if tea will help battle cancer. The best results have been seen in the laboratory. EGCG, the powerful antioxidant most abundant in green tea, inhibits cancer in a number of ways in lab experiments. It binds to free radicals and neutralizes them before they can damage healthy cells. It also seems to slow, and even reduce, the size of tumors in some animal models. There's also evidence that EGCG reduces the growth of new blood cells that would feed tumors, at least in lab experiments. And it seems that EGCG can inhibit the production of COX-2, an enzyme produced by tumors that causes inflammation and can lead to further tumor growth. Laboratory studies are a first step, but the findings aren't always replicated in human studies. Studies of people who drink green, black, or oolong tea don't always show a clear-cut benefit. Some studies show a protective effect against certain cancers, while others do not. The differences in these studies may be explained by the variations in overall diet, environment, and genetics among the study groups. And since no two pots of tea are exactly the same, the participants aren't taking in a standardized number of flavonoids. Many human studies are based on surveys that ask participants to recall what they ate and drank, how often, and how much. These can be quite unreliable, leading to false study conclusions. The type of cancer is also a significant factor in determining tea's protective and healing benefits. Some cancers appear to be more greatly impacted by tea than others.

Tea for Diabetes Control

Observational studies conducted in large populations have shown that people who consume green tea have a lower risk of developing type 2 diabetes, the most common form of diabetes among adults. A couple of smaller studies suggest that black and oolong teas may be preventive as well. But to date the findings from intervention studies in humans are mixed. One 2005 study in Japan followed 66 patients with diabetes or borderline diabetes who took either 500 mg of powdered green tea polyphenols daily or no green tea pills for two months. They found no clear effect of green tea polyphenols on blood glucose levels or on insulin resistance. But a 2003 study of Taiwanese adults with diabetes found that drinking oolong tea combined with taking hypoglycemic drugs may be an effective treatment for type 2 diabetes. The participants were on blood glucose-lowering medications and were given either six cups of oolong tea or water per day. After one month, the glucose levels of those given the oolong tea were significantly reduced compared to those given water alone.

Immune System

Green tea may help prevent rheumatoid arthritis or other immune system disorders. Researchers have been prompted to look at green tea's potential because the incidence of these health problems

AN INCONVENIENT TEA TRUTH

To get the maximum number of antioxidants from tea, you have to brew it yourself. According to the U.S. Department of Agriculture, instant teas and bottled teas contain very few antioxidants. Manufacturers are not required to put this information on their labels. The good news? You can use the convenient tea bag to brew your own and still get plenty of antioxidants.

is significantly lower in China and Japan, the two leading consumers of green tea. In 2003, scientists at Case Western Reserve University treated cartilage tissue cultures with green tea extract and found that the treated cells released less of the enzyme associated with arthritis, joint inflammation, and cartilage deterioration than cells that were not treated with the extract. Doctors already recommend a diet rich in fruits, vegetables, and fish for arthritis patients because antioxidants and omega-3 fatty acids can reduce the symptoms of arthritis. It's likely that green tea offers at least some of the healthful benefits of these foods.

Tea may also boost the body's power to fight bacterial infections. A small study at Brigham and Women's Hospital in 2003 found that patients who drank 20 ounces of black tea per day for two weeks had stronger resistance to infections than did a similar group of coffee drinkers. In fact, the immune system's output of an infection-fighting substance called interferon gamma was doubled or tripled. Researchers noted that the amino acid responsible for the effect, L-theanine, is also present in green and oolong teas.

Minding Your Memory

In ancient China, green tea was thought to provide mental clarity, and now evidence of that is turning up in laboratory studies. Experiments on mice and rat brain cells show that green tea antioxidants seem to prevent the formation of an Alzheimer's-related protein, beta-amyloid, which accumulates in the brain as plaque and leads to memory loss. This finding has been duplicated in a number of other cell-culture experiments. In one of these types of studies the antioxidants in black tea also were protective, although not as much as those found in green tea.

In humans, green tea has been associated with a lower risk of dementia and memory loss. A Japanese study published in 2006 in the *American Journal of Clinical Nutrition* surveyed more than 1,000 people older than age 70. Those who drank two or more cups a day of green tea were half as likely to develop dementia and memory loss as those who drank fewer than two cups per week. This effect was much weaker for black and oolong teas.

Tea Is Not for Everyone

If you are anemic or have an iron deficiency, drinking tea within an hour or two of eating foods containing iron may make these conditions worse. The pigments in tea and coffee, called tannins, bind to the iron and interfere with its absorption. People who are allergic to caffeine or tannins should also avoid tea, as it can cause skin rashes and hives. In fact, there have been a handful of studies documenting severe allergies to green tea, especially among people who work in the tea processing industry. People who take certain blood-thinning drugs, also called anticoagulants, such as warfarin (*Coumadin*), need to be cautious about drinking too much green tea. Green tea contains vitamin K, which affects blood clotting. It is not necessary for people on these drugs to avoid green tea entirely. However, large quantities of green tea (eight cups per day or more) may decrease their effectiveness. People taking anticoagulants should also avoid taking high doses of dietary supplements containing green tea leaves in their powdered form, unless approved by their doctor. Green tea leaves contain a lot of vitamin K; in fact, they have more than five times the amount found in black tea leaves.

Research into the possible health effects of tea is ongoing and will continue to interest researchers in the years to come. Hidden within tea's leaves there may be clues that could lead to new treatments or even cures for diseases in the future. In the meantime, enjoy tea for the simple joy of its taste and aroma and know that in doing so, you may be protecting your health as well.

ANCIENT REMEDIES

The Greeks and Romans put olives to good use. People in both of these ancient civilizations used olive oil to counteract poisons and to treat open wounds, insect bites, headaches, and stomach and digestive problems.

OLIVE OIL

Olive oil works to keep hearts healthy, may reduce inflammation and the risk of certain cancers, and might even play a role in controlling diabetes and weight.

Clearly, there is more to it than great taste!

A diet that is rich in olive oil has enhanced the health of people living in the Mediterranean region for thousands of years. Within the past century, however, olive oil's benefits have been scientifically investigated, acknowledged, and proclaimed across the globe.

Chronic diseases and conditions that are caused, in part, by unhealthy foods and sedentary lifestyles plague many societies today, especially those in the Western world. The good news is olive oil may help with the worst of them, including heart disease, hypertension (high blood pressure), inflammation, cancer, diabetes, and the various problems associated with obesity.

Healthy Fat

These conditions take many years to develop, but inactivity and consumption of too much solid fat (saturated fat and trans fat) greatly increase your chances of having to deal with them. However, olive oil and diets rich in monounsaturated fat may help combat the development of some chronic conditions.

There are two important polyunsaturated fats that are essential for human health, but the body cannot make them. This means we must get them from the foods we eat. These two essential fatty acids are alpha-linolenic acid, an omega-3 fatty acid, and linoleic acid, an omega-6 fatty acid. The body gets both from olive oil. Omega-3 oils are the healthiest. They are part of a group of substances called prostaglandins that help keep blood cells from sticking together, increase blood flow, and reduce inflammation. This makes omega-3 oils useful in preventing cardiovascular disease as well as inflammatory conditions, such as arthritis.

Omega-6 oils are healthy, too, but they are not quite as helpful as omega-3's. Omega-6's can help form prostaglandins that are similarly beneficial to the ones produced by omega-3's, but they can also produce harmful prostaglandins. The unfavorable prostaglandins increase blood-cell stickiness and promote cardiovascular disease, and they also appear to be linked to the formation of cancer. To encourage your body to make beneficial prostaglandins from omega-6 oils, you should decrease the amount of animal fat you eat. Too much animal fat tends to push your body into using omega-6 oils to make the unfavorable prostaglandins rather than the helpful ones.

Get Heart Help from Olive Oil

Research abounds regarding the benefits of monounsaturated fat. Other studies are showing that the potent phytochemicals (those substances in plants that may have health benefits for people) in olive oil—specifically, a group called phenolic compounds—appear to promote good health. Studies have shown that a phytochemical in olive oil called hydroxytyrosol "thins" the blood. Other phytochemicals reduce inflammation of the blood vessels, prevent oxidation of fats in the bloodstream, protect blood vessel walls, and dilate the blood vessels for improved circulation. Olive oil also boosts heart health by keeping a lid on cholesterol levels. It lowers total cholesterol, LDL cholesterol, and triglyceride levels. Some studies show that it does not affect HDL cholesterol; others show that it slightly increases HDL levels.

Cooling Inflammation

Inflammation within the body may occur in response to cigarette smoking or eating large amounts of saturated fat and trans fat. In overweight or obese people, excess fat from fat cells can float through the bloodstream and cause inflammation. Although inflammation can help the body, it can also hurt.

Certain dietary fats cause more of an inflammatory response than others. Trans fat and the saturated fat in animal foods stimulate inflammation. To a smaller extent, polyunsaturated fat in foods such as safflower oil, sunflower oil, and corn oil triggers inflammation, as well. Again, this is where olive oil helps. Olive oil's phytonutrients—in this case phenolic compounds called squalene, beta-sitosterol, and tyrosol—don't cause inflammation: they reduce it.

What Is Inflammation?

Inflammation is the immune system's first line of defense against injury and infection. When an injury occurs, such as a simple cut on the finger, a set of events takes place within your body that forms a blood clot, fights infection, and begins the healing process. Inflammation is painful because blood vessels dilate upstream of the injury to bring more blood and nutrients to the injured area, but they constrict at the injury site. These actions result in fluids from the bloodstream pooling in tissue around the injury, which causes swelling and pressure that stimulate nerves and cause pain.

In some individuals, the immune system gets confused and begins to view some of the body's own healthy cells as "foreign invaders." It therefore directs an immune response—complete with inflammation—at healthy tissues, harming or even destroying them. This misdirected attack results in what's called an autoimmune disorder ("auto" meaning self). Rheumatoid arthritis and certain types of thyroid disease are autoimmune disorders. Asthma, too, is the result of inflammation gone awry.

When inflammation continues unabated for long periods of time, damage can occur in organs, such as the colon, or in blood vessels. Indeed, chronic inflammation within the body is looking more and more like a serious contributor to cardiovascular (heart and blood vessel) disease. Inflammation may damage the inner lining of blood vessels, which encourages plaque deposits to form. Inflammation may also cause plaque in arteries to break off and travel downstream, where it can become lodged and stop blood flow to a crucial artery that provides oxygen to important body parts, such as your heart or brain. When this happens, a heart attack or stroke (respectively) can occur.

Yet another condition that appears to be linked to inflammation is type 2 diabetes, the most common form of diabetes that affects millions of Americans. Having excess body fat seems to increase inflammation. As inflammation increases, so does insulin resistance. As insulin resistance increases, blood glucose levels rise and the risk of type 2 diabetes skyrockets.

Scientists have discovered that inflammation can be reduced with low daily doses of aspirin or other nonsteroidal anti-inflammatory drugs (NSAIDs), which in turn appear to reduce the risk of diseases caused by inflammation. Fortunately, not only does olive oil not prompt the kind of inflammation other types of fat can, it actually has some ability to reduce inflammation, thanks to those helpful phytochemicals (squalene, beta-sitosterol, and tyrosol). So consuming olive oil on a regular basis may help decrease the risk of conditions linked to inflammation.

Oleocanthal

An article published by Philadelphia researchers in the September 2005 issue of *Nature* identified a compound in olive oil called oleocanthal that has anti-inflammatory action. Their studies revealed that this compound can act like ibuprofen and other anti-inflammatory medications. Olive oils differ widely in the amount of

WHAT COLORS SAY

Olive oils made from unripe, green olives have a light- to deep-green color. Oils made from ripe olives tend to be a golden- or light-yellow color. The color of olive oil is not an indicator of quality in relationship to culinary uses; however, if you're looking to get the most polyphenols from your olive oil, choose one with golden or yellow tints because they come from ripe olives and may contain more healing compounds.

oleocanthal they possess. To get an idea of how oleocanthal-rich your olive oil of choice is, researchers suggest taking a sip of the oil to "see how strongly it stings the back of the throat." The stronger the sting, the more oleocanthal the oil contains.

Fifty grams (nearly a quarter of a cup of olive oil) provides the same amount of anti-inflammatory action as 10 percent of the standard adult dose of ibuprofen. Obviously, eating enough olive oil to equal a whole dose of ibuprofen is not a practical way to decrease your inflammation and pain. But consuming a moderate amount of olive oil daily—in place of most of the other fat you typically consume—over the long term may lessen chronic inflammation throughout the body and bloodstream. It might even somewhat diminish asthma and rheumatoid arthritis symptoms.

Storage

Because of olive oil's high monounsaturated fat content, it can be stored longer than most other oils—as long as it is stored properly. Oils are fragile and need to be treated gently to preserve their healthful properties and to keep them from becoming a health hazard full of nasty free radicals.

When choosing your storage location, remember that heat, air, and light are the enemies of oil. These elements help cre-

ate free radicals, which eventually lead to excessive oxidation and rancidity in the oil that will leave a bad taste in your mouth. Even worse, oxidation and free radicals contribute to heart disease and even cancer.

Rancidity can set in long before you can taste it or smell it. Rotten oils harm cells and use up precious antioxidants. Even though rancid oil doesn't pose a health risk, the less you consume, the better for you.

The best storage containers for olive oil are made of either tinted glass (to keep out light) or a nonreactive metal, such as stainless steel. Avoid metal containers made of iron or copper because the chemical reactions between the olive oil and those metals create toxic compounds. Avoid most plastic, too; oil can absorb noxious substances

FREEZING OLIVE OIL

If you need to store your oil for a long period of time, stick it in the freezer. Believe it or not, olive oil freezes well, retaining its health properties and flavor. However, its complex mixture of oils and waxes prevent it from freezing at exactly 32 degrees Fahrenheit. Folk wisdom says you can tell the quality of an olive oil from the temperature at which it freezes, but this is not true.

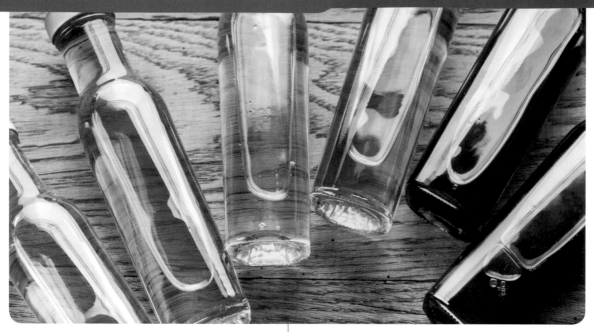

such as polyvinyl chlorides (PVCs) out of the plastic. Containers also need a tight cap or lid to keep out unwanted air.

Temperature is also important in preventing degradation of olive oil. Experts recommend storing the oil at 57 degrees Fahrenheit, the temperature of a wine cellar. Aren't lucky enough to have a wine cellar? A room temperature of about 70 degrees Fahrenheit will be fine. If your kitchen is routinely warmer than that, you can refrigerate the oil. In fact, refrigeration is best for long-term storage of all olive oils except premium extra-virgin ones. Consider keeping small amounts of olive oil in a sealed container at room temperature. This way, your olive oil is instantly ready to use. Keep the rest in the refrigerator, but remember that refrigerated olive oil will solidify and turn cloudy, making it difficult to use. Returning it to room temperature restores both its fluidity and color.

Another option is to store olive oil in a wide-mouth glass jar in the refrigerator. Even though it solidifies, you can easily spoon out any amount you need. A clear jar is fine because it's dark inside the refrigerator most of the time.

If you don't want to refrigerate your olive oil, keep it in a dark, cool cupboard away from the stove or other heat-producing appliances. Olive oil connoisseurs recommend storing premium extra-virgin olive oils at room temperature. If refrigerated, condensation could develop and adversely affect their flavor. Refrigeration does not affect the quality or flavor of other olive oils.

Olive oil will keep well if stored in a sealed container in a cool, dark cupboard for about one year. If unopened, the oil may keep for as long as two years.

Older Isn't Better

Unlike wine, oil does not improve with age. As olive oil gets older, it gradually breaks down, more free oleic acid is formed, the acidity level rises, and flavor weakens. Extra-virgin oils keep better because they have a low acidity level to start with, but you should use lower-quality oils within months because they start out with higher acidity levels. As oil sits on your shelf, its acidity level rises daily, and soon it is not palatable.

You'll get the best quality and flavor from your olive oil if you use it within a year of pressing. Olive oil remains at its peak for about two or three months after pressing, but unfortunately, few labels carry bottling dates or "use by" dates, let alone pressing dates.

More is at issue than flavor: Research shows the nutrients in olive oil degrade over time. In a study that appeared in the May 2004 issue of the *Journal of Agriculture and Food Chemistry,* Spanish researchers tested virgin olive oil that had been stored for 12 months under perfect conditions. What they found was quite surprising: After 12 months, many of the oil's prime healing substances had practically vanished. All the vitamin E was gone, as much as 30 percent of the chlorophyll had deteriorated, and 40 percent of the beta-carotene had disintegrated. Phenol levels had dropped dramatically, too.

Usage

Olive oil helps carry the flavor of foods and spices, provides a pleasing feel in the mouth, and satisfies the appetite. Liberal use of it will enhance both savory and sweet dishes without guilt because of its wonderful health-boosting properties (although if you're trying to lose weight, you may not want to overdo it, because like all fats, it provides nine calories per gram). Virgin and extra-virgin oils are best used uncooked or cooked at low to medium temperatures. Refined and olive-oil-grade oils are the choices for high-heat uses, such as frying.

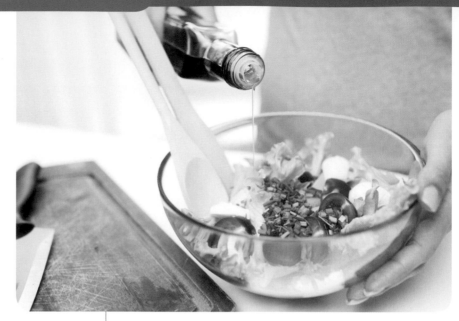

An oil's smoke point is the temperature at which it smokes when heated. Any oil is ruined at its smoke point and is no longer good for you. If you heat an oil to its smoke point, carefully discard it and start over. Olive oil has a higher smoke point than most other oils (about 400 degrees Fahrenheit). Refined olive oils have a slightly higher smoke point (about 410 degrees Fahrenheit).

Here are some ways to use olive oil:

- Drizzle it over salad or mix it into salad dressing.

- Use in marinades or sauces for meat, fish, poultry, and vegetables. Oil penetrates nicely into the first few layers of the food being marinated.

- Add at the end of cooking for a burst of flavor.

- Drizzle over cooked pasta or vegetables.

- Use instead of butter or margarine as a healthy dip for bread. Pour a little olive oil into a small side dish and add a few splashes of balsamic vinegar, which will pool in the middle and look very attractive.

- For an easy appetizer, toast baguette slices under the broiler, rub them lightly with a cut clove of garlic, and add a little drizzle of olive oil.

- Replace butter with olive oil in mashed potatoes or on baked potatoes. For the ultimate mashed potatoes, whip together cooked potatoes, roasted garlic, and olive oil; season to taste.

- Make a tasty, heart-healthy dip by mixing cooked white beans, garlic, and olive oil in a food processor; season to taste with your favorite herbs.

Baking with Olive Oil

Most people don't think of using olive oil when baking, but it's actually a great way to get more monounsaturated fat and polyphenolic compounds in your diet. Choose the lite, light, or mild type of olive oil for baking, especially savory breads and sweets such as cakes, cookies, and other desserts. Because of the filtration these types of oils have undergone, they withstand high-heat cooking methods.

Substituting olive oil for butter dramatically reduces the amount of fat—especially saturated fat—in your baked goods. And of course, olive oil does not contain any of butter's cholesterol. You'll also use less fat—you can substitute three tablespoons of olive oil for a quarter-cup of butter. (Check your cookbook for substituting advice.) The product still turns out as expected, but with 25 percent less fat, fewer calories, and even more heart-healthy nutrients.

HEALING HERBS, VITAMINS, AND SUPPLEMENTS

Nutritional supplements range from the familiar vitamins and minerals to herbal remedies. Each can support good health and help prevent and treat various disorders. Remember, though, that just because a substance is natural does not mean it can't be harmful. In excess or under certain conditions, many natural substances can be toxic. That's why it's important not to self-diagnose. If you are using prescription medications, tell all your doctors about every supplement and medication you take. Decide on a dosage that is safe for you in consultation with your health care providers.

A common perception is that because vitamins, herbs, and other supplements are natural, they are automatically gentler and don't cause side effects like drugs do. That's not always the case, however. Some do have a mild effect and don't appear to cause adverse reactions. But herbal preparations are not as strictly regulated in the United States as are medications, so it's difficult to be sure

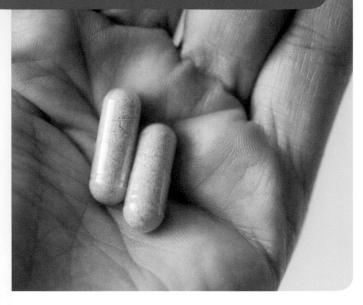

that you're getting the ingredients and doses that you pay for. In addition, some herbs can cause dangerous side effects, especially when taken at high doses, taken for longer than recommended, or taken while you're using medication.

In the rest of this chapter, we'll look first at some specific vitamins, and that at herbs and supplements, that may boost your immune health.

VITAMIN A AND CAROTENOIDS

In the case of vitamin A, the eyes have

- Follow recommended doses. More does not mean better.
- Stop using a remedy if you experience any side effects.
- Do not collect herbs from the wild.
- Only buy over-the-counter remedies if the packet states what it contains.
- Don't take herbal remedies if you are pregnant or nursing.
- Follow the directions on the package.

it. The essential nutrient vitamin A, or retinol, plays a vital role in vision. Carotenoids, the colorful plant pigments some of which the body can turn into vitamin A, are powerful protectors against cancer and heart disease.

Functions

The most clearly defined role of vitamin A is the part it plays in vision, especially the ability to see in the dark. Vitamin A deficiency is a major cause of blindness in the world.

Vitamin A is also important for normal growth and reproduction—especially proper development of bones and teeth. Animal studies show that vitamin A is essential for normal sperm formation, for growth of a healthy fetus, and perhaps for the synthesis of steroid hormones.

Another important, but misunderstood, role of vitamin A involves preserving healthy skin—inside and out. Taking extra vitamin A won't make your sagging skin suddenly beautiful, but a deficiency of it will cause major skin problems.

TOO LITTLE, TOO MUCH

Symptoms of vitamin A deficiency include night blindness, dry and rough skin, and susceptibility to infectious diseases. Symptoms of vitamin A toxicity, or overdose, include hair loss, joint pain, nausea, bone and muscles soreness, diarrhea, and enlarged liver and spleen.

Furthermore, an adequate vitamin A intake ensures healthy mucous membranes of the gastrointestinal and respiratory tracts. In this way, vitamin A helps the body resist infection.

Sources

Both animal and plant foods have vitamin A activity. Retinol, also called preformed vitamin A, is the natural form found in animals. Carotenoids, found in plants, are compounds that the body can convert to vitamin A. These precursor to vitamin A are sometimes called provitamin A. Bright-orange beta-carotene is the most important carotenoid for adequate vitamin A intake because it yields more vitamin A than alpha- or gamma-carotene.

Some carotenoids, such as lycopene, do not convert to vitamin A at all. Lycopene, the orange-red pigment found in tomatoes and watermelon, is still of value, however, because it's an antioxidant even more potent than beta-carotene. The other carotenoids are also valuable antioxidants.

Liver is the single best food source of vitamin A. However, many experts recommend eating liver only once or twice a month because of the toxic substances it can contain. Environmental pollutants tend to congregate in an animal's liver. Egg yolk, cheese, whole milk, butter, fortified skim milk, and margarine are also good sources of vitamin A. Be careful, though, as all these foods—except fortified skim milk—are also high in total fat and saturated fat, and all except margarine are high in cholesterol.

Because of the high fat and cholesterol content of most vitamin A-rich foods, as well as the potential for overdosing, it is recommended that you do not look to these sources to fulfill your need for vitamin A. Instead, rely on the provitamin plant forms of carotenoids, which do not accumulate in your liver.

Orange and yellow fruits and vegetables have high vitamin A activity because of the carotenoids they contain. Generally, the deeper the color of the fruit or vegetable, the higher the concentration of carotenoids. Carrots, for example, are especially good sources of beta-carotene and, therefore, are high in vitamin A value. Green, leafy vegetables such as spinach, asparagus, and broccoli also contain large amounts of carotenoids, but their intense green pigment, courtesy of chlorophyll, masks the tell-tale orange-yellow color.

Most other carotenoids, such as alpha- and gamma-carotene, plus cryptoxanthin and beta-zeacarotene have less vitamin A activity than beta-carotene, but offer ample cancer prevention. Some carotenoids, such as lycopene, zeaxanthin, lutein, capsanthin, and canthaxanthin are not converted into vitamin A in the body. But again, they are powerful cancer fighters, prevalent in both fruits and vegetables.

Therapeutic Value

In addition to treating deficiency syndromes, vitamin A has several potential preventive and therapeutic uses. Vitamin A is important "medicine" for the immune system. It keeps skin and mucous membrane cells healthy. When membranes are healthy they stay moist and resistant to cell damage. The moistness inhibits bacteria and viruses from "putting down stakes" and starting infectious diseases. Healthy cells are also resistant to cancers. Vitamin A fights cancer by inhibiting the production of DNA in cancerous cells. It slows down tumor growth in established cancers and may keep leukemia cells from dividing.

This vitamin is particularly helpful in diseases caused by viruses. Measles, respiratory viruses, and even human immunodeficiency virus (HIV), the virus that causes AIDS, may retreat in the presence of vitamin A. Blood levels of vitamin A are often low in people with viral illnesses. After receiving additional amounts of this vitamin, the body is able to mount its defenses, often resulting in a quicker recovery.

Carotenes, like vitamin A, support immune function, but in a different way. They stimulate the production of special white blood cells that help determine overall immune status. They improve the communication between cells, too, which results in fewer cell mutations. White blood cells attack bacteria, viruses, cancer cells, and yeast. Women with high levels of carotenes in their blood tend to have fewer incidences of vaginal yeast infections.

VITAMIN B$_6$: PYRIDOXINE

Many researchers speculate that Americans don't get enough vitamin B$_6$. Although there's no evidence of severe deficiency, many nutritionists believe the usual intake of the vitamin falls well below the RDA, perhaps causing borderline deficiency. Certain food dyes, especially FD&C yellow #5 and medications such as dopamine, penicillin, and isoniazid, interfere with vitamin B$_6$ so the body ends up with less of the nutrient available for use. Widespread use of these B$_6$ an-

tagonists may be the underlying problem behind many of the health conditions that respond favorably to supplementation of the vitamin.

Functions

It's called simply vitamin B$_6$, but researchers discovered early on that this vitamin is not one substance, but three: pyridoxine, pyridoxamine, and pyridoxal. All three have the same biological activity and all three occur naturally in food.

Pyridoxine functions mainly by helping to metabolize protein and amino acids. Though not directly involved in the release of energy, like some other B vitamins, pyridoxine helps remove the nitrogen from amino acids, making them available as sources of energy. Because of its work with proteins, it plays a role in the synthesis of protein substances such as muscles, antibodies, and hormones. It also helps out in the production of red blood cells, neurotransmitters (chemical messengers), and prostaglandins that regulate certain metabolic processes. This vitamin gets together with more than 60 enzymes in the body, working to get many functions accomplished.

Sources

Vitamin B_6 is in all foods, in one form or another. Plant foods are generally high in pyridoxine, while pyridoxamine and pyridoxal are more common in foods of animal origin. All three forms of vitamin B_6—pyridoxine, pyridoxamine, and pyridoxal—appear to have the same biological activity.

Protein foods, meats, whole wheat, salmon, nuts, wheat germ, brown rice, peas, and beans are good sources. Vegetables contain smaller amounts, but if eaten in large quantities, they can be an important source. Even though pyridoxine is lost when grains are milled to make flour, manufacturers do not regularly add it back to enriched products, except some highly fortified cereals.

Therapeutic Value

Entire books have been written on the therapeutic uses of vitamin B_6; it has been used to treat more than 100 health conditions.

Pyridoxine has a role in preventing heart disease. Without enough pyridoxine, a

TOO LITTLE, TOO MUCH

If people are marginally deficient in vitamin B_6, they may be more susceptible to carpal tunnel syndrome. Carpal tunnel syndrome is characterized by pain and tingling in the wrists after performing repetitive movements or otherwise straining the wrist on a regular basis. A lack of the vitamin may play a role in sensitivity to monosodium glutamate (MSG), a flavor enhancer. This sensitivity can cause headaches, pain and tingling of the upper extremities, nausea, and vomiting. In both of these syndromes, supplementation of pyridoxine alleviates symptoms only when people were deficient in the vitamin to begin with.

Despite being water-soluble, pyridoxine is toxic in high doses, causing reversible nerve damage to the extremities. Doses of 200 mg or more for an extended period of time can trigger tingling and numbness in the hands and feet. When dosage levels are reduced, symptoms disappear.

compound called homocysteine builds up in the body. Homocysteine damages blood vessel linings, setting the stage for plaque buildup when the body tries to heal the damage. Vitamin B_6 prevents this buildup, thereby reducing the risk of heart attack. Pyridoxine lowers blood pressure and blood cholesterol levels and keeps blood platelets from sticking together. All of these properties work to keep heart disease at bay.

Prone to kidney stones? Pyridoxine, teamed up with magnesium, prevents the formation of stones. It usually takes about three months of supplementation to make blood levels of these nutrients sufficient to keep stones from forming.

Vitamin B_6 has long been publicized as a cure for premenstrual syndrome (PMS). Study results conflict as to which symptoms are eased, but some of the claims include reduced bloating and relief of breast pain. The exception to this controversy seems to be premenstrual acne flare, a condition in which pimples break out about a week before a woman's period begins. There is strong evidence that pyridoxine supplementation, starting ten days before the menstrual period, prevents most pimples from forming. This effect is due to the vitamin's role in hormone regulation. Skin blemishes are typically caused by a hormone imbalance, which vitamin B_6 helps to regulate.

Mental depression is another condition which may result from low vitamin B_6 intake. Because of pyridoxine's role in serotonin and other neurotransmitter production, supplementation often helps depressed people feel better, and their mood improves significantly. It may also help improve memory in older adults. Women who are on hormone-replacement therapy or birth control pills often complain of depression and are frequently deficient in vitamin B_6. Supplementation improves these cases, too.

Low intakes of pyridoxine can slow down the immune system. Several different immune components become rather sluggish in the absence of adequate vitamin B_6, making a person more susceptible to diseases.

People with asthma can benefit from pyridoxine supplements. Clinical studies of the nutrient show that wheezing and asthma attacks decrease in severity and frequency during vitamin B_6 supplementation. Anyone with breathing difficulties who is taking the drug theophylline may want to consider supplementation with this vitamin. Theophylline interferes with vitamin B_6 metabolism. Supplementation not only normalizes blood levels but also helps limit the headaches, anxiety, and nausea that often accompany theophylline use.

The nausea and vomiting that frequently accompany the early stages of pregnancy sometimes respond to pyridoxine treatment.

VITAMIN C: ASCORBIC ACID

When you hear the word *vitamin C,* you may instinctively think of the common cold. For that you can thank Linus Pauling and his 1970 book, *Vitamin C and the Common Cold.* In it, Pauling recommended megadoses of vitamin C to reduce the frequency and severity of colds. The book triggered a sales boom for vitamin C that is still going strong. It also prompted nutritionists to begin a series of carefully designed studies of the vitamin and its functions.

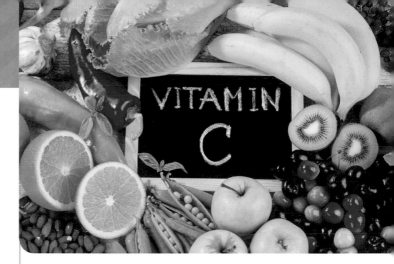

Today, some people still swear by vitamin C. Researchers have found little proof of its effectiveness against catching the common cold, but there is evidence to suggest it can reduce the severity and length of a cold.

Functions

A major function of vitamin C is its role as a cofactor in the formation and repair of collagen—the connective tissue that holds the body's cells and tissues together. Collagen is a primary component of blood vessels, skin, tendons, and ligaments. Vitamin C also promotes the normal development of bones and teeth. Furthermore, it's needed for amino acid metabolism and the synthesis of hormones, including the thyroid hormone that controls the rate of metabolism in the body. Vitamin C also aids the absorption of iron and calcium.

These days, vitamin C is heralded for its antioxidant status. It prevents other substances from combining with free oxygen radicals by tying up these free radicals of oxygen themselves. In this role, vitamin C protects a number of enzymes involved in functions ranging from cholesterol metabolism to immune function. It destroys harmful free radicals that damage cells and can lead to cancer, heart disease, cataracts, and perhaps even aging. Vitamin C rejuvenates its cousin antioxidant, vitamin E.

min C in significant amounts since they are widely consumed by Americans on a regular basis. Though cooking destroys some of the vitamin, you can minimize the amount lost if the temperature is not too high and you don't cook them any longer than necessary.

Rose hips from the rose plant—used to prepare rose-hip tea—are rich in vitamin C. Fruit juices, fruit juice drinks, and drink mixes may be fortified with vitamin C at fairly high levels.

Sources

Of course, the famed citrus fruits—oranges, lemons, grapefruits, and limes—are excellent sources of vitamin C. Other often overlooked excellent sources of vitamin C are strawberries, kiwifruit, cantaloupe, and peppers. Potatoes also supply vita-

TOO LITTLE, TOO MUCH

The classic vitamin C deficiency disease is scurvy. Early signs of the disease are bleeding gums and bleeding under the skin, causing tiny pinpoint bruises. The deficiency can progress to the point that it causes poor wound healing, anemia, and impaired bone growth. Since only 10 mg of vitamin C is needed daily to prevent scurvy, the disease is rarely seen today. In very large amounts, it can have adverse effects such as cramps, diarrhea, and destruction of vitamin B_{12}, and decreased copper absorption.

More than with any other vitamin except folate, vitamin C is easy to destroy. The amount in foods falls off rapidly during transport, processing, storage, and preparation. Bruising or cutting a fruit or vegetable destroys some of the vitamin, as does light, air, and heat. Still, if you cover and refrigerate orange juice, it will retain much of its vitamin C value, even after several days. For maximum vitamin value, it's best to use fresh, unprocessed fruits and vegetables whenever possible.

Therapeutic Value

Vitamin C is the most popular single vitamin. Besides taking it to treat colds, people pop vitamin C capsules hoping that it will cure numerous ailments. There is now scientific evidence to support some of that hope.

Scientifically controlled studies using vitamin C for colds show that it can reduce the severity of cold symptoms, acting as a natural antihistamine. The vitamin may be useful for allergy control for the same reason: It may reduce histamine levels. By giving the immune system one of the important nutrients it needs, extra vitamin C can often shorten the duration of the cold as well. However, studies have been unable to prove that megadoses of the vitamin can actually prevent the common cold.

As an important factor in collagen production, vitamin C is useful in wound healing of all types. From cuts and broken bones to burns and recovery from surgical wounds, vitamin C taken orally helps wounds to heal faster and better. Applied topically, vitamin C may protect the skin from free radical damage after exposure to ultraviolet (UV) rays.

Vitamin C makes the headlines when it comes to cancer prevention. Its antioxidant properties protect cells and their DNA from damage and mutation. It supports the body's immune system, the first line of defense against cancer, and prevents certain cancer-causing compounds from forming in the body. Vitamin C reduces the risk of getting almost all types of cancer. It appears that this nutrient doesn't directly attack cancer that has already occurred, but it helps keep the immune system nourished, enabling it to battle the cancer.

VITAMIN E: TOCOPHEROL

Vitamin E is not actually a single compound, but rather several different compounds, all with vitamin E activity. One, d-alpha-tocopherol, has the greatest activity. Other compounds with vitamin E activity are beta-tocopherol, gamma-tocopherol, and delta-tocopherol.

Functions

Vitamin E functions as an antioxidant in the cells and tissues of the body. It protects polyunsaturated fats and other oxygen-sensitive compounds such as vitamin A from being destroyed by damaging oxidation reactions. Vitamin E's antioxidant properties are also important to cell membranes. For example, vitamin E protects lung cells that are in constant contact with oxygen and white blood cells that help fight disease. A deficiency of vitamin E thus weakens the immune system.

But the benefits of vitamin E's antioxidant role may actually go much further. Vitamin E may protect against heart disease and may slow the deterioration associated with aging. Critics scoffed at such claims in the past, but an understanding of the importance of vitamin E's antioxidant role may be beginning to pay off.

Sources

Oils and margarines from corn, cottonseed, soybean, safflower, and wheat germ are all good sources of vitamin E. Generally, the more polyunsaturated an oil is, the more vitamin E it contains, serving as its own built-in protection. Fruits, vegetables, and whole grains contain less. Refining grains reduces their vitamin E content, as does commercial processing and storage of food. Cooking foods at high temperatures also destroys vitamin E. So a polyunsaturated oil is useless as a vitamin E source if it's used for frying. Your best sources are fresh and lightly processed foods, as well as those that aren't overcooked.

These days, it's difficult to get much vitamin E in the diet because of cooking and processing losses and because of the generally reduced intake of fat. Moreover, the current emphasis on monounsaturated fats, such as olive oil or canola oil, rather than vitamin E-containing polyunsaturated fats, further decreases our intake of vitamin E. Monounsaturated fats have other benefits for the heart, though, so you shouldn't stop using olive and canola oils. It is important to find other sources of vitamin E. Besides, the fewer polyunsaturated fats you eat, the less vitamin E you need, so your requirements may be lower if you switch to olive or canola oils.

Therapeutic Value

As an antioxidant with a powerful punch, vitamin E helps prevent cancer, heart disease, strokes, cataracts, and possibly some of the signs of aging. Vitamin E protects artery walls and keeps the "bad" low-density lipoprotein (LDL) cholesterol from being oxidized. Oxidation of LDL cholesterol marks the beginning of clogged arteries. Vitamin E also keeps the blood thin by preventing blood platelets from clumping together. High levels of vitamin E in the body greatly decrease the risk of heart attack and stroke. If these events do occur and vitamin E is

TOO LITTLE, TOO MUCH

No obvious symptoms accompany a vitamin E deficiency, making it hard to detect. A brownish pigmentation of the skin may signal the problem, but only a blood test can confirm that vitamin E levels are too low. When diseases of the liver, gall bladder, or pancreas reduce intestinal absorption, a mild deficiency of vitamin E can result. A diet of processed foods that's very low in fat might also cause a deficiency.

Too much vitamin E might delay blood clotting, possibly causing an increased risk of stroke or uncontrolled bleeding in the event of an accident. Because of this possibility, people on anticoagulant therapy (blood thinners) should not take large doses of vitamin E.

low, they are likely to be more serious since there are insufficient amounts of this protective nutrient to combat the oxidative damage that occurs.

A dynamic cancer fighter, vitamin E protects cells and DNA from damage that can turn cancerous. It reduces the

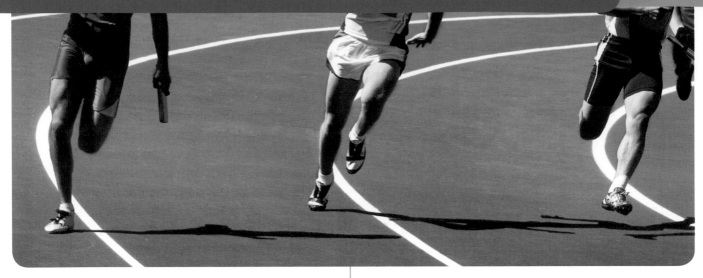

growth of tumors while enhancing immune function and preventing precancerous substances from being turned into carcinogens. Studies with mice show that vitamin E applied to the skin may help prevent skin cancer resulting from exposure to ultraviolet radiation.

This humble nutrient keeps the nervous system healthy by protecting the myelin sheaths that surround nerves. It also appears to prevent mental degeneration due to aging, possibly even including Alzheimer disease.

Athletes need to get adequate amounts of vitamin E. The body's own metabolism creates free radicals during excessive aerobic exercise. Vitamin E reserves make sure these free radicals don't get out of hand and cause trouble. Vitamin E therapy also treats claudication—pains in the calf muscles that occur at night or during exercise.

There are many more uses of vitamin E that science is only beginning to investigate. This helpful vitamin will probably continue to make the news every so often as we learn more.

IRON

The average human body contains only a few grams of iron, but without this vital mineral our tissues would not be able to get oxygen, and life would be impossible.

Functions

Most of the body's iron resides in the hemoglobin of red blood cells—the pigment that makes these blood cells appear red. Hemoglobin carries oxygen to cells and transports carbon dioxide from cells. Iron is also essential to enzymes involved in energy release, cholesterol metabolism, immune function, and connective-tissue production.

Sources

Good sources of iron include liver and other meats, whole grains, shellfish, green leafy vegetables, and nuts. Iron is one of the nutrients commonly added to enriched cereals and bread. According to recent research, soybean hulls (not the whole soybean) contain a very absorbable form of iron. In the future, these hulls may be used to fortify other foods.

Cooking in iron pots adds iron to the foods prepared in them. This is especially true of acidic foods such as tomatoes.

Absorption of iron is notoriously poor; only about 10 percent of iron consumed is absorbed. The iron in meat—called

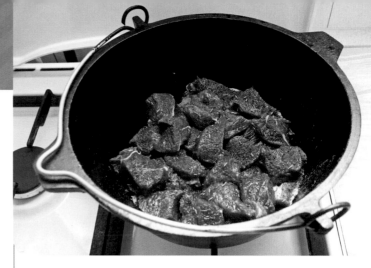

heme iron—is absorbed better than the iron found in vegetables—*nonheme* or *organic* iron. Meat, fish, poultry, and vitamin C all increase iron absorption. Eating any of these at a meal increases the amount of iron absorbed from most other foods eaten during that meal. Coffee, tea, whole soybeans, and whole grains, however, all reduce the amount of iron absorbed from foods when eaten at the same meal.

About Iron Deficiency

Iron deficiency is the most common cause of anemia. Headaches, shortness of breath, weakness, fatigue, cognitive impairment, heart palpitations, and sore tongue are some of the symptoms. For people who are anemic, even mild exercise can cause chest pain. Mild iron deficiency even without anemia may cause learning problems in school children and reduce work productivity in adults.

Pica, a desire to eat nonfood substances such as clay, chalk, ashes, or laundry starch (none of which contains iron) sometimes accompanies iron deficiency. This abnormal craving may be an underlying factor contributing to the anemia or the result of a deficiency.

Long-term use of aspirin can cause bleeding in the lining of the stomach. The blood loss may lead to iron deficiency. Aspirin coated with a special material reduces irritation to the stomach lining. Drinking plenty of water when you take aspirin also helps.

Young children fed mostly milk, with few other foods, can develop a milk-induced iron-deficiency anemia. Milk contains little iron and in very large quantities may actually promote irritation and bleeding in the stomach. Anemia can result from this loss of blood coupled with low intake.

The normal acidity of the stomach helps promote iron absorption in the intestine. Chronic use of antacids decreases the acidity of the stomach, reducing the amount of iron absorbed. This sets the stage for a deficiency.

Pregnant women, children, women with heavy menstruation, and frequent blood donors are at greater risk for iron deficiency.

Therapeutic Value

Some people, especially those on medications such as fluoxetine (Prozac), may experience a condition called restless legs syndrome. These patients are agitated and move constantly. Even with no anemia present, iron supplementation of 200 mg ferrous sulfate three times per day greatly reduced the symptoms in elderly patients.

Iron may help increase an athlete's endurance. As part of hemoglobin, iron carries oxygen to muscles; it also helps enzymes that are involved in how the body adapts to exercise. In addition, many athletes may be marginally deficient in iron because of foot strike hemolysis—repeatedly striking the feet on a hard surface, as in jogging, leads to destruction of blood cells. The body needs iron to replace the destroyed red blood cells.

Sufficient iron keeps the brain supplied with oxygen and improves learning ability. If children don't get enough iron from birth to age four, they consistently do poorer in school and on IQ tests than their non-iron-deficient counterparts. This phenomena carries through their school years; the iron-deficient children never quite catch up to their peers.

Pregnancy is a time when special attention must be given to adequate iron intake. Inadequate amounts may lead to premature delivery and low-birth-weight infants—both linked to health problems for the newborn.

Adequate iron levels are also important for optimal immune function. However, many invading bacteria also need iron, so supplementing iron during an infection may not be a good idea. Better to have adequate iron stores as a routine measure.

Iron is very valuable to the body, but doses larger than the RDA are never indicated except in the case of mild or severe deficiency. To treat an iron deficiency, you need iron supplements in conjunction with an iron-rich diet. Once a person develops iron deficiency anemia, it may take up to one year of iron supplementation to replenish body stores.

Iron in all ferrous forms is better absorbed than is ferric iron. Ferrous succinate is the best-absorbed form of non-heme iron. When you read labels on iron supplements, check for the amount of elemental iron. That's what's important. For example, the label may state, "Each tablet provides 200 mg of ferrous fuma rate, which yields 67 mg of elemental iron."

Cautions to Consider

Some people don't tolerate iron supplements well and may develop side effects such as heartburn, nausea, stomachache, constipation, or diarrhea. Taking the supplement with food can eliminate or minimize these symptoms. Also look for supplements that are formulated to be "nonconstipating." You can gradually work up to the desired dose or divide the high dose into several small doses. Don't worry if your stool appears dark. It's just some of the unabsorbed iron.

In healthy people, the intestines control the amount of iron that's absorbed. The body increases its rate of iron absorption if reserves are low. And when the body becomes saturated with iron, the rate decreases. If the intestines do not or cannot properly perform this regulatory function—as can happen from excessive and prolonged alcohol intake—the body can absorb toxic quantities.

A certain percentage of the population suffers from *hemochromatosis,* a hereditary disease in which the body absorbs too much iron and deposits it in body tissues. Hemochromatosis most often affects men. Because men usually get enough iron, experts advise that men avoid the extra iron in some supplements and cereals. Although it's difficult to accurately assess whether a person has hemochromatosis, serum ferritin is a good indicator.

Symptoms of this condition only appear after significant and irreversible damage occurs. They include weakness, weight loss, change in skin color, abdominal pain, loss of sex drive, and the onset of diabetes. Heart, liver, and joints may also become impaired. In particular, the extra iron creates free radicals that damage blood vessels and cholesterol, paving the way for heart disease. Cancer cells, too, like extra iron; cancer patients should avoid supplementation, as the extra iron can cause the cancer cells to grow even more rapidly.

Iron poisoning is the most common accidental poisoning in young children.

Iron tablets may be coated with sugar to mask their taste, and if allowed access to them, children will eat them like candy. *IRON CAN BE FATAL TO CHILDREN. All supplements should be kept out of the reach of children.*

SELENIUM

Selenium is found in all body tissues, with the highest concentrations found in the kidneys, liver, spleen, pancreas, and testicles.

Functions

Selenium functions as an antioxidant as part of the enzyme glutathione peroxidase. It helps prevent cell damage from free radicals that form when oxygen attacks, or oxidizes, fats and other compounds. Selenium supports the immune system, helping it function optimally, and it appears to have antiviral properties, killing viruses under laboratory conditions.

Sources

The Brazil nut is such a super source, don't eat more than a few at a time. Good sources also include meat and fish. The amount found in grains depends on the selenium content of the soil in which they were grown. Some studies show that the soil levels of selenium have been severely depleted in many parts of the United States. However, a typical American diet generally provides the RDA of selenium without the use of supplements.

Therapeutic Value

Studies suggest that selenium may have anticancer properties by working as an antioxidant along with vitamin E and in the enzyme glutathione peroxidase. These actions protect cells and prevent DNA damage, which can lead to the development of malignancies. Selenium

TOO LITTLE, TOO MUCH

Severe deficiency of selenium affects heart function, but a deficiency is hard to detect because vitamin E can substitute for selenium in some of its functions, thus masking the classic symptoms. Hair loss, nail changes, fatigue, nerve problems in the extremities, and nausea and vomiting are hallmarks of selenium toxicity.

may also help prevent cancer by inhibiting cell replication. It seems most useful in fighting digestive tract cancers.

These same antioxidant properties account for selenium's role in preventing heart disease and strokes. Glutathione peroxidase prevents free radical damage of artery walls and the oxidation of low-density lipoprotein (LDL) cholesterol. This mineral is also helpful after a heart attack or stroke, possibly preventing reoccurrence.

Glutathione peroxidase enhances the immune system, assisting white blood cells. People with cataracts have less selenium in their eye fluids. Glutathione peroxidase's antioxidant activities work to prevent this disabling eye disease.

Inflammatory arthritis, such as the rheumatoid type, may be managed by selenium supplementation. Selenium is involved in the inflammation process, helping to regulate substances that control inflammation, while glutathione peroxidase attacks the tissue-damaging free radicals that result from inflammation.

Selenium may also help prevent skin cancer. Oral and topical selenium helped mice exposed to ultraviolet light avoid skin cancer. Some experts feel this could be helpful for humans as well.

ZINC

Most zinc resides in our bones. The rest of this trace mineral turns up in skin, hair, and nails. In men, the prostate gland contains more zinc than any other organ.

Functions

Zinc is a part of more than 200 different enzyme systems that aid the metabolism of carbohydrates, fats, and proteins. One of these enzymes, superoxide dismutase, serves as an antioxidant in cells. Zinc is also part of the hormone insulin, helping transport vitamin A from its storage site in the liver to where it is used in the body.

Sources

Oysters contain much more zinc than any other food. Meat, poultry, eggs, and liver are also rich sources. Two servings of animal protein daily provide most of

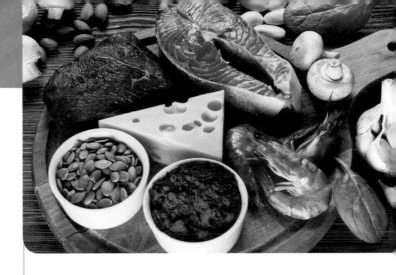

the zinc a healthy person needs. Whole grains contain fair amounts of zinc, but they also harbor phytates, substances that tie up zinc and other minerals and prevent absorption. Yeast counteracts the action of phytates, so eating whole-grain breads still affords good nutrition.

Therapeutic Value

As a cofactor in more than 200 enzymes, adequate zinc intake is critical for good health. Zinc boosts the immune system and enhances the activity of white blood cells. Optimal immune function is vital for avoiding colds, flu, cancer, and infectious diseases in general. Zinc supplements before and during an illness can help the body put up

a better fight. Zinc lozenges dissolved slowly in the mouth help to resolve a cold and sore throat. Viruses responsible for illness are inhibited by zinc; they're unable to replicate. Zinc can be of help to older adults, whose immune systems tend to slow with age.

The prostate gland in men requires adequate zinc for proper functioning. Inadequate intake is one of the causes of prostate enlargement. This is called benign

TOO LITTLE, TOO MUCH

Zinc deficiency has serious effects, including: retarded growth and sexual development, delayed wound healing, a low sperm count, depressed immune system (making infections more likely), reduced appetite, and altered sense of taste and smell.

As with other minerals, taking too much zinc can have the opposite of the effect desired. Excessive amounts will depress immune function and create other deficiencies and complications, such as skin outbreaks, high blood cholesterol levels, anemia, and scurvylike symptoms. Excess zinc can also cause a copper deficiency.

prostatic hyperplasia. It is not linked to prostate cancer, but it can still cause urination problems. Zinc supplementation is known to help reduce an enlarged prostate. This mineral is also critical to sperm production and motility as well as male hormone regulation in general, helping to improve male fertility.

Zinc has been used successfully to treat acne. It is active in hormone regulation and occurs in high quantities in the skin. Taken at 30 mg per day for three months, zinc will likely help to diminish acne's severity.

Supplements of zinc may help prevent heart disease. The mineral strengthens the integrity of the cells that line the walls of the arteries, making them more resistant to the damage that can start the process of plaque buildup. Its role in the enzyme superoxide dismutase, which is an antioxidant, also helps keep arteries in good shape.

Older adults may benefit from additional zinc intake. Tinnitus, the constant and annoying ringing in the ears that often plagues older adults, may be linked to zinc-dependent enzymes. Supplementation of zinc can lessen or stop the ringing. Many seniors suffer from macular degeneration, a condition that leads to vision loss. Zinc supplements may help prevent progression to loss of sight.

Zinc may also be beneficial in diabetes, viral infections, and certain skin conditions.

Many experts suspect that marginal zinc intakes are common in the United States. As many as 90 percent of elderly Americans may take in suboptimal amounts of zinc. Why? As we cut back on meat, we cut out an important source of zinc. Low-calorie diets also tend to be low in zinc.

Vegetarian diets, especially vegan diets that do not contain any animal products, may promote a zinc deficiency. If vegetarians eat whole-grain breads made with yeast, they absorb zinc better, because yeast breaks down the phytates in whole grains. Unleavened bread, such as pita and flat bread, contains intact phytates that tie up zinc, preventing its absorption.

Pumpkin seeds are a good vegetarian source.

Strict vegetarians might consider a supplement. A multimineral supplement that contains iron isn't the best choice because iron interferes with zinc absorption.

Infections, injuries, or other physical sources of stress can cause zinc loss in the urine, and people with these conditions may want to consider supplementation as an answer.

Supplements might be able to help a great many conditions. If you supplement zinc for more than several weeks, it should be accompanied by copper to avoid copper deficiency; consult your health care provider for the correct ratio.

ALGAE PRODUCTS

Some species of algae are full of beneficial nutrients. Two common ones are chlorella, a green algae, and spirulina, a blue-green algae. Both are single-celled organisms that live in fresh water. Once

TOO LITTLE, TOO MUCH

There are no dosage guidelines available for algae products. Algae appears to be safe and nonallergenic. Testing has not revealed any biogenic toxins or toxic metals at significant levels, and no toxicity has been noted in animal studies for spirulina.

harvested, they are dried and made into supplements.

Sources

Algae is either collected from lakes, where it grows naturally, or it is grown synthetically. Occasionally naturally growing algae can be contaminated by toxin-producing algae that start growing alongside it. Some of these unwanted algae produce substances that are toxic to the liver. Therefore, "cultured" algae grown in synthetic conditions may be safer than naturally growing algae.

Therapeutic Value

Algae is rich in amino acids, vitamins, minerals, carotenoids and gamma-linolenic acid (GLA)—a fatty acid that helps promote health. Spirulina contains an easily absorbed form of iron.

Both chlorella and spirulina are often used as supplements during weight loss to decrease appetite, help shed pounds, and improve physical and mental energy. Research, however, has yet to bear out these claims.

Chlorella has exhibited strong antitumor properties in animals. It contains superoxide dismutase—a powerful antioxidant—so it can prevent cell mutations, which are often the first step in the development of cancer. It may have other anticancer powers as well.

Chlorella decreases inflammation. In animal research, chlorella reduced the amount of cholesterol the body absorbed and stimulated the excretion of bile

acids, which is one way the body gets rid of cholesterol.

Studies from Japan show that spirulina can jump-start the immune system. It increases the number of antibodies and several types of white blood cells.

Spirulina may play a role in heart health. It prevents artery spasm and pushes the body to make substances that dilate blood vessels. Spirulina effectively keeps the bloodstream from getting too "thick" and clotting internally. This algae prompts the body to make certain prostaglandins—substances that reduce blood pressure, lower blood levels of "bad" low-density lipoprotein (LDL) cholesterol, and increase levels of "good" high-density lipoprotein (HDL) cholesterol. Spirulina prevents the formation of unfavorable prostaglandins that have the opposite effects as those just mentioned.

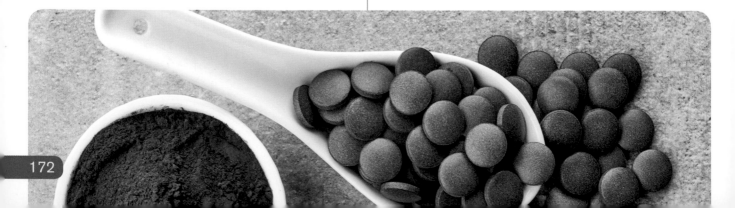

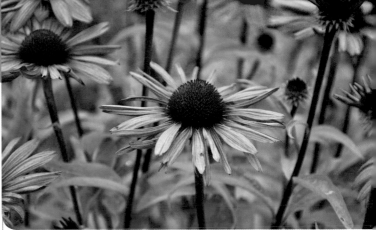

ECHINACEA

The roots and sometimes the leaves of this beautiful sunflower family member (*Echinacea purpurea*) make an important medicine used widely to treat colds, flu, bronchitis, and all types of infections.

Therapeutic Value

This showy perennial was used by the Native Americans and adopted by the early settlers as a medicine. Members of the medical profession in early America relied heavily on echinacea, but it fell from favor with the advent of pharmaceutical medicine and antibiotics. Many physicians are rediscovering the benefits of echinacea today. Many forms of echinacea are available to choose from.

Long used for infectious diseases and poor immune function, echinacea extractions are also used today to help treat cancer, chronic fatigue syndrome, and AIDS. Research has shown echinacea stimulates the body's natural immune function. It also increases both the number and the activity of white blood cells, raises the level of interferon, and stimulates blood cells to engulf invading microbes. Echinacea also increases the production of substances the body produces naturally to fight cancers and disease.

Besides its use as an immune stimulant, echinacea is recommended for individuals with recurring boils and as an antidote for snake bites.

CAUTION

Due to their medicinal value, many tons of the roots are sold annually; thus, echinacea species are disappearing from the wild. It might be best to grow your own echinacea or purchase it from a reputable herb source that cultivates its own herbs and not from people who harvest echinacea from its native habitat.

Echinacea is considered quite safe, even at high and frequent doses. However, frequent use of echinacea may mask the symptoms of a more serious underlying disease. If you have any persistent condition, be sure to consult a physician.

Preparation and Dosage

Echinacea is not terribly tasty in a tea. For this reason, echinacea is most often taken as tincture or as pills. However, teas and tinctures appear to be more effective than the powdered herb in capsules. If you take the capsules, first break them open and put them in a little warm water; then drink the water. Most herbalists recommend large and frequent doses at the onset of a cold, flu, sinus infection, bladder infection, or other illness.

For acute infection: Take one dropper full of tincture every one to three hours, or 1 to 2 capsules every three to four hours for the first day or two; then reduce the dosage.

For a chronic infectious problem: Take echinacea three times a day for several weeks and then abstain for several weeks before continuing again.

GARLIC

Garlic's résumé would read something like this: cholesterol lowerer, blood pressure reducer, blood sugar balancer, cancer combatant, fungus fighter, bronchitis soother, cold curer, wart remover, and immune system toner.

Therapeutic Value

With a résumé like this, it's no wonder garlic (*Allium sativum*) is so popular with advocates of herbal medicine. This member of the Lily family is one of the most extensively researched and widely used of all plants. Its actions are diverse and affect nearly every body tissue and system. Lots of people include garlic in their daily diet for health reasons, while many others eat it because they love its pungent flavor. Many thousands of acres are devoted to cultivating garlic in the United States.

As an antimicrobial, garlic seems to have a broad action. It displays antibiotic, antifungal, and antiviral properties and is reportedly effective against many flu viruses and herpes simplex type I strains (the virus responsible for cold sores). You may add garlic liberally to soups, salad dressing, and casseroles during the winter months to help prevent colds, or eat garlic at the first hint of a cold, cough, or flu. Garlic reduces congestion and may help people with bronchitis to expel mucus.

Garlic is used to treat many types of infections: Use capsules internally for recurrent vaginal yeast infections, use a garlic infusion topically as a soak for athlete's foot, or add garlic to an oil to treat middle ear infections.

This popular herb may improve immunity by stimulating some of the body's natural immune cells. Studies suggest that garlic may help prevent and treat breast, bladder, skin, and stomach cancers. One study of women in Iowa suggests that women who eat garlic may lower their risk of colon cancer. Garlic appears particularly effective in inhibiting compounds formed by nitrates, which are preservatives used to cure meat that are thought to turn into cancer-causing com-pounds within the intestines.

Garlic lowers blood pressure by relaxing vein and artery walls. This action helps keep platelets from clumping together and improves blood flow, thereby reducing the risk of stroke. Garlic also

ROASTED GARLIC

Peel two bulbs of garlic and combine in a small roasting dish with sliced red bell pepper, a grated carrot, and a small amount of peanut oil. Place underneath the broiler for two or three minutes, stir the pepper and carrot, and broil for two or three minutes more. The bulbs should become slightly browned. Eat small amounts frequently at the onset of a cold or a flu for a natural antibiotic effect.

decreases the level of LDL (low-density lipoprotein, or "bad" cholesterol).

Garlic contains a large number of rather unique sulfur-containing compounds, which are credited with many of this herb's medicinal actions. Did you ever wonder why garlic bulbs on your kitchen counter don't have a strong odor until you cut or crush them? That's because an enzyme in garlic promotes conversion of the chemical compound alliin to the odorous allicin. Allicin and other sulfur compounds are potent antimicrobials and are thought to have blood purifying and, possibly, anti-cancer effects.

The constituents in garlic also increase insulin levels in the body. The result is lower blood sugar. Thus garlic makes an excellent addition to the diet of people with diabetes. It will not take the place of insulin, anti-diabetes drugs, or a prudent diet, but garlic may help lower insulin doses.

Preparations and Dosage

Garlic is available fresh, dried, powdered, and tinctured. In health food stores, garlic appears primarily in capsule form or combined in tablets with other herbs. Since garlic's antibiotic properties depend on odorous allicin, deodorized garlic preparations are not

HOW MUCH IS TOO MUCH?

Some individuals are sensitive to garlic and cannot use it in large amounts without feeling nauseous and hot. Others don't digest sulfur compounds well, and gas and bloating result. Garlic used topically, such as in eardrops for ear infections, can irritate skin and membranes in sensitive people. If you know that too much garlic upsets your stomach, don't eat it or ingest it as a medicine. If you're not sure, use garlic cautiously at first to determine how well you tolerate it. Nursing mothers may find that ingesting too much garlic flavors breast milk, causing some infants to reject it. Other babies develop a stronger sucking reflex in response to the mother's consumption of garlic.

effective for this use. The label of such products may identify them as having a particular "allicin content," but they remain ineffective as antibiotics. Deodorized products are quite effective for lowering blood pressure and cholesterol, however. Of course, the tastiest way to get your dose of garlic is to add it liberally to your diet. Brushing your teeth or nibbling on fresh parsley after eating garlic can help keep your breath socially acceptable.

Capsules: Take 800 mg a day.

Tincture: Take 1 or 2 droppers full in a glass of water, two to four times daily. For painful ear infections, place 1 or 2 drops of warm garlic oil in the ear canal several times a day at the onset of ear pain.

Infusion for topical use: Crush a garlic bulb, and steep in 4 to 5 cups of hot water. Soak feet in the preparation for 15 to 20 minutes up to three times a day to treat athlete's foot.

GINGER

This botanical and popular spice (*Zingiber officinale*) is native to southeast Asia but is now readily available in the United States. Fresh ginger root is a staple in Asian cooking. Dried and powdered, it's used in medicine. Ginger is high in volatile oils, also known as essential oils. Volatile oils are the aromatic part of the plants that lend the flavor and aroma we associate with most culinary herbs. They are called "volatile" because as unstable molecules they are given off freely into the atmosphere.

Therapeutic Value

Ginger root powder may be useful in improving pain, stiffness, mobility, and swelling. Larger dosages of approximately 3 or 4 grams of ginger powder daily appear most effective. But powder may not be the only effective form of ginger root: One study demonstrated a response from the ingestion of lightly cooked ginger.

Ginger has also had a long history of use as an anti-nausea herb recommended for morning sickness, motion sickness, and nausea accompanying gastroenteritis (more commonly called stomach flu). As a stomach calming agent, ginger also reduces gas, bloating, and indigestion, and aids in the body's use and absorption of other nutrients and medicines. It is also a valuable deterrent to intestinal worms, particularly roundworms. Ginger may even improve some cases of constant

severe dizziness and vertigo. It may also be useful for some migraine headaches. Ginger also prevents platelets from clumping together in the bloodstream. This serves to thin the blood and reduce your risk of atherosclerosis and blood clots.

A warming herb, ginger can promote perspiration when ingested in large amounts. It stimulates circulation, particularly in the abdominal and pelvic regions, and can occasionally promote menstrual flow. If you are often cold, you can use warm ginger to help raise your body temperature.

WHEN TO AVOID GINGER

Since ginger can warm and raise body temperature slightly, it should be avoided when this is undesired, such as in someone with menopausal hot flashes.

Avoid ginger preparations for fevers that are over 104°F. Although ginger is recommended for morning sickness, those with a history of miscarriage should avoid it. Since ginger stimulates blood flow and thins the blood, promoting uterine bleeding is a concern. Some people actually become nauseous if they consume a large quantity of ginger; for others, ginger relieves nausea. It is best to use ginger cautiously at first.

When used topically, ginger stimulates circulation in the skin, and the volatile oils travel into underlying tissues. Try ginger root poultices on the chest for lung congestion or on the abdomen for gas and nausea. Powdered ginger and essential oils are the strongest form of ginger for topical use.

Preparations and Dosage

Capsules: For nausea, take 1 to 2 capsules every two to six hours. To alleviate arthritis pain, try higher dosages of 15 to 25 capsules per day.

Tea: Drink 1 or 2 cups of ginger tea to promote a warming effect. To promote actual perspiration, you'll need more.

Warming Tea Recipe

- 10 to 12 thin slices of fresh ginger root
- 4 cups of water
- Juice of 1 orange
- Juice of $\frac{1}{2}$ lemon
- $\frac{1}{2}$ cup honey or maple syrup (optional)

GINGER POULTICE FOR THROAT OR LUNG CONGESTION

Grate one whole ginger root into a bowl. Stir in $\frac{1}{4}$ tsp of cayenne oil or powder and 2 drops of essential oil of thyme. Place a liberal coat of plain oil or ointment on the area of skin to be treated. For swollen tonsils and enlarged lymph nodes in the neck, oil the neck, throat, and underside of the chin. For bronchitis and lung congestion, oil the upper chest and back. Spread the grated ginger root mixture on the skin and cover with a sheet of plastic wrap. Cover this with a heating pad or hot, moist towel. Leave in place for 15 to 30 minutes. The skin should turn red and feel warm and stimulated, but you should feel no pain with this procedure. Remove the poultice promptly if you experience any discomfort or burning. For infants and adults with sensitive skin, you may want to omit the cayenne and thyme oil and instead use plain grated ginger.

Place ginger root and water in a pan, and boil ten minutes. Strain. Add orange and lemon juices and honey. Consume as a warming tea. Several large cups consumed in a row or drunk in a hot bath can elevate the body temperature and promote perspiration. This sweating therapy may help break a fever or reduce congestion.

GINSENG

So popular is this herb that more than 50,000 people are employed worldwide in the ginseng industry. Rather than addressing specific conditions, ginseng is used to treat underlying weakness that can lead to a variety of conditions. For example, among its many uses, ginseng is recommended for people who are frequently fatigued, weak, stressed, and affected by repeated colds and flu. Ginseng is an adaptogen, capable of protecting the body from physical and mental stress and helping bodily functions return to normal.

Ginseng Varieties

The enthusiasm over ginseng began thousands of years ago in China, where the Asian species of ginseng, *Panax ginseng,* grows. So valued was China's native species, the plant was overhar-

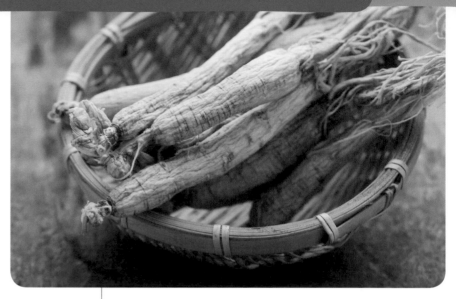

vested from the wild, causing scarcity and increased demand. A mature woods-grown root of *Panax ginseng* will sometimes fetch $1,000 or more. A mature *wild* woods-grown root of *Panax ginseng* will sometimes fetch $200,000 or more!

When a similar species, *Panax quinquefolius,* was noted in the early American colonies, tons of the plant were immediately dug and exported to China. Many American pioneers made their living digging ginseng roots from moist woodlands. As a result, ginseng has become rare in its natural habitat in the United States as well. Ginseng is now cultivated in forests or under vast shading tarps.

Many people believe the cultivated ginseng has slightly different properties than the natural wild specimens. The Asian species is said to be the superior medicine compared with the American species, but the two species have slightly different applications. The Asian *Panax ginseng* is said to be a yang tonic, or more warming, while the American *Panax quinquefolius* is said to be a yin tonic, or more cooling. Both the *ginseng* and the *quinquefolius* species are qi tonics, or agents capable of strengthening qi, our vital life force.

In traditional Chinese medicine, our vital qi is composed of two opposing forces, yin and yang. Yin and yang are dualistic opposites that churn and cycle in all life and, indeed, all matter. The yang aspect of the life forces is the bright, hot, masculine, external, dispersive, dynamic pole. The yin aspect is the dark, moist, feminine, internal, contracted, mysterious pole. All people, all plants, all matter, and yes, even all diseases have their yin and yang aspects.

Traditional Chinese medicine is very sophisticated in its observation of these phenomena, thus all botanical therapies are fine-tuned accordingly. *Panax ginseng,* for example, might be recommended to warm and stimulate someone who is weak and cold from nervous exhaustion. *Panax quinquefolius,* on the other hand, is best for someone who is hot, stimulated, and restless from nervous exhaustion and feverish wasting disease. It is good for someone experiencing a lot of stress (and subsequent insomnia). American ginseng is used in China to help people recuperate from fever and the feeling of fatigue associated with summer heat.

Therapeutic Value

Asian ginseng is used as a general tonic by modern Western herbalists as well as by traditional Chinese practitioners. It is thought to gently stimulate and strengthen the central nervous system in cases of fatigue, physical exertion, weakness from disease and injury, and prolonged emotional stress. Its most widespread use is among the elderly. It is reported to help control diabetes, improve blood pressure and heart action, and reduce mental confusion, headaches, and weakness among the elderly. Asian ginseng's affinity for the nervous system and its ability to promote relaxation makes it useful for stress-related conditions such as insomnia and anxiety. Serious athletes may benefit from the use of Asian ginseng with improved stamina and endurance. Animal and human studies have shown Asian ginseng possibly reduces the occurrence of cancer: Ginseng preparations increase production of immune cells, which may boost immune function.

Ginseng contains many complex saponins referred to as ginsenosides. Ginsenosides have been extensively studied and found to have numerous complex actions, including the following: They stimulate bone marrow production, stimulate the immune system, inhibit tumor growth, balance blood sugar, stabilize blood pressure, and detoxify the liver, among many other tonic effects. Ginseng also contains numerous other constituents, yet no one constituent has been identified as the most active. In fact, many of the individual constituents have been shown to have opposite actions. Like all plant medicine, the activity is due to the sum total of all the substances.

The Chinese consider the Asian species *Panax ginseng* a yang tonic, so it is not used in those who have what traditional Chinese medicine refers to as yang excess, or excess heat. This means that people who are warm or red in the face or have high blood pressure or rapid heartbeat should not use Asian ginseng. American ginseng is much better suited to this type of person. But conversely,

WHEN TO AVOID GINSENG

Ginseng is one of the better researched plants, and no serious toxicity has ever been reported. Due to hormonal activity, however, ginseng should be avoided during pregnancy. Some cases of hypertension are aggravated by ginseng while others are improved; consult an herbalist, naturopathic physician, or other practitioner trained in the use of herbal medicine for the use of ginseng in hypertension.

American ginseng should not be used in those who are cold or pale or in those with a slow heartbeat. Possible side effects of Asian ginseng use include, curiously, some of the symptoms it is prescribed for: hypertension, insomnia, nervousness, and irritability. Acne and diarrhea are also occasionally reported.

Seek advice from an herbalist or naturopathic physician who can determine if ginseng is appropriate for you and, if so, can recommend an appropriate dose. Due to potential hormonal activity, Asian ginseng can promote menstrual changes and breast tenderness on occasion. The side effects caused by ginseng resolve quickly once the herb is discontinued.

RED CLOVER

Have you ever taken a nip of nectar from the tiny florets of this familiar meadowland plant (*Trifolium pratense*)? The bees certainly do. Clover honey is one of the most common types of honey available, and bees visit red clover throughout the summer and fall. The edible flowers are slightly sweet. You can pull the petals

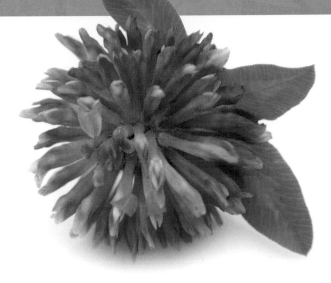

from the flower head and add them to salads throughout the summer. A few tiny florets are a delightful addition to a summer iced tea: Serve your summer guests a cup of iced mint tea with a lemon slice and five to ten tiny clover florets floating on top. You can also press the fresh florets into the icing on a summer birthday cake.

The raw greens of this plant are very nutritious, but like other members of the legume family (beans, peas), they are somewhat difficult to digest. The leaves are best enjoyed dried and in the tea form to get the nutrients and constituents without the side effects of gas and bloating common to eating legumes.

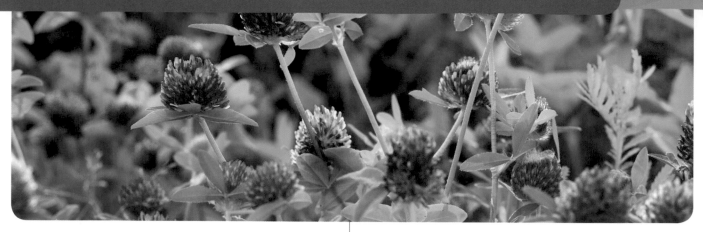

Therapeutic Value

Red clover's constituents are thought to stimulate the immune system. (It has been a traditional ingredient in many formulas for cancer.) Red clover has also been used to treat coughs and respiratory system congestion, since it also contains resin. Resinous substances in plants have expectorating, warming, and antimicrobial action. Red clover also contains the bloodthinning substance coumarin. Coumarin is not unique to red clover and is found in many other plants, including common grass. In fact, the pleasant sweet smell of freshly cut grass is due to the coumarin compounds. People on anticoagulant drugs such as Coumadin should be cautious of using red clover since the blood may become too thin. There has been much research on compounds related to coumarin, and much of the hormonal effects of red clover is attributed to these compounds. Here's why: When a hormone molecule is released from various organs, it travels through the bloodstream until it binds to a cell membrane, called a hormone receptor, that is able to receive it. If a compound in a plant is close enough to the shape of the body's natural hormone molecule, it may also bind to the receptor on a cell membrane. What this means is that some substances in plants produce the same effects in humans as some hormones. Coumarins in red clover are able to bind to estrogen—and possibly other—receptors. They appear to have substantial hormonal effects.

It has been noted for some time that male sheep that graze on large quantities of red clover eventually develop a diminished sperm count. (There is, however, no evidence that red clover causes low sperm counts in human males. A human could not eat enough to affect sperm counts.) It is also common for female sheep to develop uterine fibroids. Fibroids are a noncancerous tumor; their growth within the uterine wall in humans is thought to be associated with too much estrogen in the system. It may be that the coumarins in red clover have an estrogenic effect when consumed as a staple part of the diet. We have much yet to learn about coumarins, but it seems logical that they may prove useful in conditions associated with very low estrogen levels (menopause, chronic miscarriage, some cases of infertility) and should be avoided in cases of estrogen excess (uterine fibroids, endometriosis, breast cancer). Red clover has been a traditional folk therapy for infertility and chronic miscarriage, both of which can be due to insufficient estrogen.

WHEN TO AVOID IT

Those with abnormally low platelet counts, those using anticoagulant drugs, and those with clotting defects should avoid red clover preparations. Do not consume red clover before surgery or childbirth, as it may impair the ability of the blood to clot. Red clover is believed to promote the growth of uterine fibroids in sheep, but whether this is true for humans is unknown. There is also some concern that red clover may stimulate cancers that are fed by estrogen, such as some breast and uterine cancers. Until more is known, it may be best for patients with hormonally influenced cancers or uterine fibroids to avoid red clover.

On the whole, red clover is considered very safe, and little effect aside from occasional gas is noticed from drinking the tea. The mild anticoagulant effect and the hormonal effects, however, are undesirable for some individuals.

Preparations and Dosage

Tea: You may drink several cups of red clover tea a few times a week for general purposes. Drink several cups daily for two to ten weeks for a medicinal effect.

Tincture: Take 2 to 4 droppers full (1 to 2 teaspoons) daily.

AN OUNCE OF PREVENTION

We've talked about lifestyle changes such as diet, exercise, and stress management that can boost your immune system. But there are some other relatively straightforward steps you can take to stay healthy.

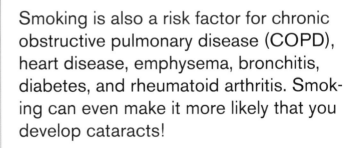

STOP SMOKING

At this point it is widely known that smoking has deleterious effects on your health. People often think, however, mostly of lung cancer. This is understandable, since smoking is responsible for approximately 90% of lung cancer deaths. But smoking can also cause cancer in other parts of your body, including the trachea, esophagus, larynx, liver, and bladder.

The CDC estimates that, "If nobody smoked, one of every three cancer deaths in the United States would not happen."

Smoking is also a risk factor for chronic obstructive pulmonary disease (COPD), heart disease, emphysema, bronchitis, diabetes, and rheumatoid arthritis. Smoking can even make it more likely that you develop cataracts!

Quitting smoking is, of course, easier said than done. What works for one person will not work for another, and someone may have to try several methods before one sticks. And, while some smokers can quit "cold turkey," most will need support—from their doctors, from their families, and perhaps through a program. There are multiple medications now available for helping smokers quit smoking. For the technologically savvy, there are even online communities and mobile apps!

FILTER IT OUT

Unfortunately, what you can't see can hurt you. Dust and particulates in the air, and contaminants in your water, may be affecting your health.

Tap water, for example, is safer in some areas than others. Depending on the contaminants of your water, you may benefit from a water filter. Some municipalities send out a report on water quality periodically. You can also buy your own relatively inexpensive water testing kits from a home improvement store. If you install a filter, make sure to check first about what maintenance is involved and how often filters need to be changed—if you aren't changing filters accordingly to schedule, you may give yourself a false sense of ease about your water.

Air purifiers are often recommended household with members who have allergies or asthma, but they may be helpful for other households too. You can buy a HEPA (high-efficiency particulate air) filter that's compatible with your home's HVAC system; it works by trapping particulates in a fine mesh. Just make sure to change it according to the recommended schedule. There are also small portable devices. Again, look for something with a HEPA filter. Check for information on room size as well, to make sure you're buying one that isn't too small for your living area.

WEAR SUNSCREEN

In 1997, *Chicago Tribune* columnist Mary Schmich wrote a widely-circulated essay giving advice to graduates that famously included the line, "Wear sunscreen." It's good advice, preventing both short-term pain and long-term problems!

A sunburn is one of the most common hazards of the great outdoors. The unappealing and painful lobster look results when the amount of exposure to the sun exceeds the ability of the body's protective pigment, melanin, to protect the skin. What makes sunburn different from, say, a household iron burn? The time factor. A sunburn is not immediately apparent. By the time the skin starts to become red, the damage has been done. Pain isn't always instantly noticeable, either.

You may feel glowing after two hours sitting poolside without sun protection. But just wait awhile. You'll change your tune (not to mention color) when the pain sets in, typically 6 to 48 hours after sun exposure. Like household burns, sunburns are summed up by degree. Mild sunburns are deep pink, punctuated by a hot, burning sensation. Moderate sunburns are red, clothing lines are prominent, and the skin itches and stings. Severe sunburns result in bright red skin, blisters, fever, chills, and nausea.

Being burned to a crisp can lead to serious consequences later in life. In fact, one severe, blistering sunburn during childhood doubles your chances of developing malignant melanoma, a deadly form of skin cancer, or other types of skin cancer such as basal cell and squamous cell carcinomas. If cancer doesn't frighten you, then the specter of developing premature wrinkling and age spots just might.

Obviously, covering up and applying a waterproof sunscreen with a high SPF (sun protection factor) is the best way to prevent sunburn.

Ways of the Rays

Here on earth we're exposed to two types of ultraviolet rays: UVA and UVB rays. Unlike visible light, these rays are shorter in wavelength, are higher in energy, and fall outside the visible spectrum (so you can't see what's hitting you). When these high-energy rays strike your unsuspecting skin, they generate free radicals, which can damage DNA.

UV ray damage can be short-term (a painful burn) or long-term (premature aging of the skin and skin cancer). So what's the difference between UVA and UVB rays?

UVA: Ultraviolet A

- a longer wavelength
- penetrates the deep layers of the skin and produces free radicals
- linked to premature aging of the skin
- can pass through window glass in cars, houses, and office buildings

UVB: Ultraviolet B

- a shorter wavelength
- doesn't penetrate deeply into the skin
- can cause significant damage to DNA
- the primary cause of sunburn and skin cancer
- cannot pass through windows

VACCINATIONS

They're not always pleasant—who appreciates a shot?—but a bit of unpleasantness can forestall far worse consequenc-

SUNBURN DO'S AND DON'TS

- Avoid being out in the sun between the hours of 10 A. M. and 3 P. M., when the sun's rays are the strongest.

- Don't think you're protected if the skies are cloudy. Damaging rays aren't inhibited by clouds, and you can still get burned. So wear sun protection or cover up even when it's cloudy.

- Use a waterproof sunscreen if you'll be swimming or if you'll be sweating a lot. And be sure to reapply the sunscreen frequently (follow the directions on the label).

- If you're taking any medications, be sure to check about side effects from sun exposure. Some medications, such as tetracycline, cause a rash on areas exposed to the sun.

es. Currently, the CDC recommends a schedule of childhood vaccines to prevent against chickenpox, diphtheria, *Haemophilus influenzae* type B (which can lead to meningitis and pneumonia), hepatitis A and B, influenza, measles, mumps, pertussis (whooping cough), polio, pneumococcus (which can lead to meningitis), rotavirus, rubella, and tetanus. These vaccines are given during early childhood, up to 6 years old. In preteen and teen years, there is an additional set of recommended vaccines to prevent tetanus, diphtheria, pertussis, human papillomavirus, and meningococcal disease. It is also recommended that preteens and teens, like everyone else, get a flu shot every year.

In recent years there has been some controversy over childhood vaccinations because of speculation that the vaccines may be linked to autism. Some parents have avoided vaccinating their children, or delayed and spaced out vaccinations, as a result. However, scientists have conducted extensive studies and have concluded that there is no evidence to support that link. Another idea is that it's better for children to develop immunity naturally, by getting a disease and building up resistance to it. While natural immunity can be stronger than that produced by a vaccine, the risks can be quite great if complications should develop. The concept of widespread vaccinations also ties in to the idea of herd immunity—that is, we rely on a certain

ACRONYM ALERT

The TDAP vaccine protects against tetanus, diphtheria, and pertussis. In addition to the childhood vaccination schedule, it's recommended that adults receive a booster shot for tetanus/diphtheria every 10 years, and that pregnant women receive the TDAP vaccine between 27 and 36 weeks.

percentage of the population being immune to contagious diseases in order to limit its spread. When vaccination levels in a population go below a certain percentage, there can be more outbreaks of a disease—which can be especially devastating for any people who have compromised immune systems, who could not be vaccinated. We have seen more measles outbreaks in recent years, for example.

The Flu Vaccine

You hoped you got the shots over with when you were a kid—but there are some recommended vaccinations for adults, too. It can be easy to forget about them;

as adults, we tend to go to the doctor when something specific is wrong, and it can be easy for vaccines to fall off the radar. So here are a few reminders:

It's recommended that everyone over 6 months of age get a flu shot every year. Unfortunately, you can still get the flu, even if you've gotten a flu shot. Each year, vaccinations are developed based on what viruses are circulating, and the vaccination is a better match for some strains of the virus than others. The flu vaccine can also prevent complications if you do get sick.

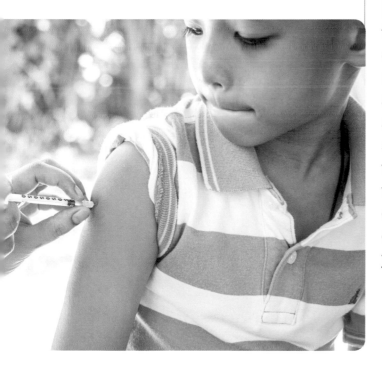

SPECIAL CONSIDERATIONS FOR SENIORS

In addition to the flu vaccine, it is recommended that adults over 60 discuss with their doctor getting vaccines against pneumococcal disease and shingles, as vulnerability increases with age.

Travelers Beware

Visitors traveling to other countries will want to look up recommended vaccines for the area to which they are traveling. For example, a typhoid vaccine or yellow fever may be recommended if those diseases are prevalent. The rabies vaccine may be recommended for people who are doing outdoors trips or working with animals. In other areas, a polio booster shot may be recommended even if you were vaccinated as a child. The CDC's web site offers information recommended vaccines for each country, depending on your destination, the type of travel you're doing, and your own health.

GETTING OVER IT QUICKLY

No matter how well you tend your health, sometimes you will get sick. In this chapter we'll look at common ailments and some basic household remedies that will ease symptoms and bolster your immune system to help you get through them as quickly and painlessly as possible.

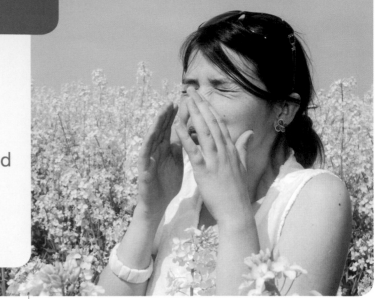

ALLERGIES

Allergies can be called a haywire response of the immune system. Normally, the immune system guards against intruders it considers harmful to the body, such as certain viruses and bacteria. That's its job. However, in allergic people, the immune system goes a bit bonkers. It overreacts when you breathe, ingest, or touch a harmless substance. The benign culprits triggering the overreaction, such as dust, pet dander, and pollen, are called allergens.

The body's first line of defense against invaders includes the nose, mouth, eyes, lungs, and stomach. When the immune system reacts to an allergen, these body parts make great battlegrounds. Symptoms include runny nose; sneezing; watery, swollen, or red eyes; nasal congestion; wheezing; shortness of breath; a tight feeling in the chest; difficulty breathing; coughing; diarrhea; nausea; headache; fatigue; and a general feeling of misery. Symptoms can occur alone or in combination.

What Causes Allergies?

Blame your genes. The tendency to become allergic is inherited, and allergies typically develop before age 30. What you become allergic to is based on what substances you are exposed to and how often you are exposed to them.

Generally, the more you are exposed to an allergen, the more likely it is to trigger a reaction. Unfortunately, there is no cure for allergies. But there are ways to ease your long-suffering sinuses and skin.

From the Cupboard

Baking soda. One-half cup baking soda poured into a warm bath is an old New England folk remedy for soothing hives. Soak for 20 to 30 minutes.

Tea. Allergy sufferers throughout the centuries have turned to hot tea to provide relief for clogged-up noses and irritated mucous membranes. One of the best for symptom relief is mint tea, which has been used by the Chinese to treat allergies since the seventh century. Mint's benefits extend well beyond its delicious smell. Mint's essential oils act as a decongestant, and substances within the mint contain anti-inflammatory and mild antibacterial constituents.

From the Freezer

Ice. Wrap a washcloth around ice cubes and apply them to your sinuses for instant relief and refreshment.

From the Refrigerator

Milk. Milk does the body good, especially when it comes to hives. Wet a cloth with cold milk and lay it on the affected area for 10 to 15 minutes.

Wasabi. If you're a hay fever sufferer and sushi lover combined, this remedy will please. Wasabi, that pale-green, fiery condiment served alongside California rolls, is a member of the horseradish family. Anyone who has taken too big a dollop of wasabi or plain old horseradish knows how it makes sinuses and tear ducts spring into action. That's because allyl isothiocyanate, a constituent in wasabi, promotes phlegm flow and has antiasthmatic properties. The tastiest way to get in those allyl isothiocyanates is by

MINT TEA RECIPE

Place $\frac{1}{2}$ ounce dried mint leaves in a 1-quart jar. Fill two-thirds of the jar with boiling water and steep for five minutes (inhale the steam). Let cool, strain, sweeten if desired, and drink.

slathering horseradish on your sandwich or plopping wasabi onto your favorite sushi. The last, harder-to-swallow option is to purchase grated horseradish and take ¼ teaspoon during an allergy attack.

From the Spice Rack

Basil. To help ease an allergic reaction or hives, try dousing the skin with basil tea, a traditional Chinese folk remedy. Basil contains high amounts of an anti-allergic compound called caffeic acid. Place 1 ounce dried basil leaves into 1 quart boiling water. Cover and let cool to room temperature. Use the tea as a rinse as often as needed.

Salt. Nasal irrigation, an effective allergy-management tool that's done right at the sink every morning, uses a mixture of salt water to rid the nasal passages of mucus, bacteria, dust, and other gunk, as well as to soothe irritated passageways. All you need is 1 to 1 ½ cups lukewarm water (do not use softened water), a bulb (ear) syringe, ¼ to ½ teaspoon salt, and ¼ to ½ teaspoon baking soda. Mix the salt and baking soda into the water and test the temperature. To administer, suck the water into the bulb and

squirt the saline solution into one nostril while holding the other closed. Lower your head over the sink and gently blow out the water. Repeat this, alternating nostrils until the water is gone. Nasal irrigation isn't a pretty sight, yet it works wonders on sore noses and rids the passages of unwanted stuff. Always make sure to use distilled, not tap, water, and a clean syringe.

From the Stove

Steam. Breathing steam refreshes and soothes sore sinuses, and it helps rid the nasal passages of mucus. While it takes some time, it will make you feel wonderful! Boil several cups of water and pour into a big bowl (or a plugged sink). Place your head carefully over the bowl and drape a towel over yourself. Breathe gently for 5 to 10 minutes.

When you're finished breathing steam, use the hot water for a second purpose. Let the water cool until warm, saturate a washcloth, and hold it on the sinuses (to the sides of your nose, below the eyes and above the eyebrows).

More Do's and Don'ts

Pass up the milk. When allergies act up, skip that extra-large, whole-milk latte since dairy products thicken mucus. Try herbal tea instead.

Shampoo before bedtime. During pollen prime time, the hair acts as one gigantic magnet, attracting flying pollen and stray mold spores. The more hair you have, and the oilier and more elaborately styled it is, the better its collection capabilities. When you lie down, these hair hitchhikers drop onto the pillow and are quickly inhaled, causing allergy symptoms that night or the next morning. To avoid being a walking collection agency, cover your hair when out for a walk or wash it before bedtime.

Boost That Immune System

An allergy-sufferer's hardworking immune system may increase demands for certain nutrients, both to protect the body and to help rebuild defenses. Be sure your diet includes the following vitamins and minerals:

- **Vitamin A.** If you eat a well-balanced diet, you should have an ample supply.

- **Vitamin B complex.** B vitamins are found in almost every food, but the

WHEN TO CALL THE DOCTOR

You can't always tell whether what's bothering you is an allergy or an infection, intolerance, or a specific disease. So check with your doctor if you experience any of the following:

- Nasal problems that cause secondary symptoms, such as chronic sinus infections, nasal congestion, or difficulty breathing
- Symptoms that last for several months
- Inability to get relief from over-the-counter medications or unacceptable side effects, such as drowsiness, from them
- Symptoms that interfere with your ability to carry out daily activities or decrease your quality of life
- Any of these symptoms, which can be warning signs of asthma: struggling to catch your breath; wheezing and coughing, especially at night or after exercise; shortness of breath; tightness in your chest

- best sources are from fresh vegetables and meats.
- **Vitamin C.** Citrus fruits are high in vitamin C.
- **Vitamin E.** High amounts are found in vegetable oils, nuts, and seeds. Moderate amounts are in avocados, asparagus, mangoes, apples, and sweet potatoes.
- **Iron.** The best sources are meats, oysters, whole grains (including hot cereals), beans, and green vegetables.
- **Selenium.** Find this mineral in meats, seafood, and whole grains.
- **Zinc.** Meats, oysters, dairy products, and some beans have good amounts of zinc.

ANEMIA

Anemia is a condition in which your red blood cell count is so low that it can't carry enough oxygen to all parts of your body. Not having enough oxygen in the blood is like trying to drive a car with no oil. Your car may run for a while, but you'll soon end up with a burned-out engine. In the same way that oil nourishes your car's engine, oxygen provides needed nourishment for your body's tissues (organs, muscles, etc.), and if they aren't getting enough of that vital sustenance, you'll start feeling weak and tired. A short climb up the stairs will leave you breathless, and even a couple days of rest won't perk you up. If that describes how you feel, check with your doctor. If you do have anemia, you should take action as soon as possible. And you need to be sure you don't have a more serious condition.

Anatomy of Anemia

Your red blood cells are the delivery trucks of the body. They carry oxygen throughout your blood vessels and capillaries to feed tissues. Hemoglobin, the primary component of red blood cells, is a complex molecule and is the oxygen carrier of the red blood cell.

The body works very hard to ensure that it produces enough red blood cells to successfully carry oxygen but not too many, which can cause the blood to get too thick. Red blood cells live only 90 to 120 days. The liver and spleen get rid of the old cells, though the iron in the cells is recycled and sent back to the marrow to produce new cells.

When you're diagnosed with anemia it usually means your red blood cell count is abnormally low, so it can't carry enough oxygen to all parts of your body, or that there is a reduction in the hemoglobin content of your red blood cells. Anemia's not a disease in itself but instead is considered a condition. However, this condition can be a symptom of a more serious illness. That's why it's always important to check with your doctor if you think you may be anemic.

The Most Common Causes of Anemia

There are many types of anemia. Some rare types are the result of a malfunction in the body, such as early destruction of red blood cells (hemolytic anemia), a hereditary structural defect of red blood cells (sickle cell anemia), or an inability to make or use hemoglobin (sideroblastic anemia). The most common forms of anemia are the result of some type of nutritional deficiency and can often be treated easily with some help from the kitchen. These common types are:

Iron deficiency anemia. Iron deficiency anemia happens when the body doesn't have enough iron to produce hemoglobin, causing the red blood cells to shrink. And if there's not enough hemoglobin produced, the body's tissues don't get the nourishing oxygen they need. Children younger than three years of age and premenopausal women are at highest risk for developing iron deficiency anemia. Most young children simply don't get enough iron in their diet, while heavy menstrual periods are the most common cause of iron deficiency anemia in women who are premenopausal. In addition, during pregnancy a woman's blood volume increases three times, boosting iron needs. Contrary to popular belief, men and older women aren't at greater risk for iron deficiency anemia. If they do end up developing the condition, it's most often the result of an ulcer.

Vitamin B_{12} deficiency anemia. While iron deficiency anemia produces smaller than usual red blood cells, a vitamin B_{12} deficiency anemia produces oversized red blood cells. This makes it harder for the body to squeeze the red blood cells through vessels and veins. It's like trying to squeeze a marble through a straw. Vitamin B_{12}-deficient red blood cells also tend to die off more quickly than normal cells. Most people get at least the minimum amount of B_{12} that they need by eating a varied diet. If you are a vegetarian or have greatly limited your intake of meat, milk, and eggs for other health reasons, you may not get enough of the vitamin in your diet. Many older people are more at risk for vitamin B_{12} deficiency; in fact, 1 out of 100 people older than 60 years of age are diagnosed with pernicious anemia. This age group is at increased risk because they are more likely to have conditions that affect the body's ability to absorb vitamin B_{12}. Surgical removal of portions of the stomach or small intestine; atrophic gastritis, a condition that causes the stomach lining to thin; and diseases such as Crohn's can all interfere with the body's ability to absorb vitamin B_{12}.

But the most common cause of vitamin B_{12} deficiency anemia is a lack of a protein called intrinsic factor. Intrinsic factor is normally secreted by the stomach; its job is to help vitamin B_{12}. Without intrinsic factor, the vitamin B_{12} that you consume in your diet just floats out as waste. In some people, a genetic defect causes the body to stop producing intrinsic factor. In other people, an autoimmune reaction, in which the body mistakenly attacks stomach cells that produce the protein, results in a lack of intrinsic factor. A vitamin B_{12} deficiency that is caused by a lack of intrinsic factor is called pernicious anemia. Pernicious anemia can be particularly dangerous because it causes neurological problems, such as difficulty walking, poor concentration, depression, memory loss, and irritability. These can usually be reversed if the condition is treated in time. Unfortunately, in the case of pernicious anemia, the stomach cannot absorb the vitamin no matter how much B_{12}-rich food you eat. So treatment requires injections of B_{12}, usually once a month, that bypass the stomach and shoot the vitamin directly into the bloodstream.

Folic acid deficiency anemia. A deficiency of folic acid produces the same oversized red blood cells as a vitamin B_{12} deficiency. One of the most common causes of folic acid deficiency anemia is simply not getting enough in the diet. The body doesn't store up folic acid for long periods like it does many other nutrients, so if you aren't getting enough in your diet, you will quickly become deficient. Pregnant women are most at risk for folic acid anemia because the need for folic acid increases by two-thirds during pregnancy. Adequate folic acid intake is essential from the start of pregnancy because it protects against spinal defects in the fetus.

Symptoms of Anemia

Symptoms of more severe anemia include rapid heartbeat, dizziness, headache, ringing in the ears, irritability, pale skin, restless legs syndrome, and confusion. A vitamin B_{12} or folic acid deficiency may even cause your mouth and tongue to swell. These symptoms may sound scary, but the most common forms of anemia are easily treated, especially if caught early.

Symptoms of mild to moderate anemia:

- weakness
- fatigue
- shortness of breath

Symptoms of moderate to severe anemia:

- rapid heartbeat
- dizziness
- headache
- ringing in the ears
- pale skin (especially the palms of your hands), pale or bluish fingernails
- hair loss
- restless legs syndrome
- confusion

Symptom specific to severe vitamin B_{12} or folic acid deficiency anemia:

- swelling of the mouth or tongue

Symptoms specific to pernicious anemia:

- numbness, tingling
- depression and/or irritability
- memory loss

Because all but pernicious anemia are the result of a nutritional deficiency, the best ways to treat them can be found in the kitchen.

From the Cupboard

Blackstrap molasses.

Consider covering that waffle or those pancakes in a little molasses. Blackstrap molasses has long been known to be a nutritional powerhouse. Containing 3.5 mg of iron per tablespoon, blackstrap molasses has been used in folk medicine as a "blood builder" for centuries.

Dry cereal. Fix yourself a bowl of your favorite cereal (go for one without the sugar and the cartoon characters on the box), and you'll be waging a battle against anemia. These days many cereals are fortified with a nutrient punch

IRON'S ABSORPTION EQUATION

You may not be absorbing as much iron from your foods as you think. How much you absorb is dependent on two primary factors: what kind of iron is in the food and what other nutrients the food contains. There are two types of iron, heme and non-heme. Heme, found primarily in foods of animal origin, is much more easily absorbed than non-heme iron, which is found primarily in plant products. But if you eat a vitamin C-rich food or a food rich in heme iron with your non-heme iron food, your body will take in more iron.

- Sources of mostly heme iron: beef liver, lean sirloin, lean ground beef, skinless chicken, pork

- Sources of non-heme iron: fortified breakfast cereal, pumpkin seeds, bran, spinach

- Sources of vitamin B_{12} : salmon (3 ounces), beef tenderloin (3 ounces), yogurt (1 cup), shrimp (3 ounces)

- Sources of folic acid: spinach ($\frac{1}{2}$ cup), navy beans ($\frac{1}{2}$ cup), wheat germ ($\frac{1}{4}$ cup), avocado ($\frac{1}{2}$ cup), orange (1 medium) of iron, vitamin B_{12}, and folic acid. Check the label for amounts per serving, pour some milk over your flakes, and dig in.

From the Refrigerator

Beef liver. Beef liver is rich in iron and all the B vitamins (including B_{12} and folic acid). In fact, beef liver contains more iron per serving—5.8 mg per 3 ounces— than any other food. Other animal sources of iron include eggs, cheese, fish, lean sirloin, lean ground beef, and chicken.

Beets. Beets are rich in folic acid, as well as many other nutrients, such as fiber and potassium. The best way to prepare beets is to nuke 'em in the microwave. Keep the skin on when cooking, but peel before eating. The most nutrient-dense part of the beet is right under the skin.

Spinach. Green leafy vegetables contain loads of iron and folic acid. We're talking dark and green, so choose your leaves carefully. Iceberg lettuce is mostly water and is of little nutritive value. Spinach, on the other hand, has 3.2 mg of iron and 130 mcg of folic acid per $\frac{1}{2}$ cup.

More Do's and Don'ts

If you're a vegetarian or have cut way down on your intake of meats, milk, and eggs, be sure that you're getting adequate amounts of iron and vitamin B_{12} in your diet. With such a diet, you are at greater risk for nutritional deficiency anemias because iron from plant sources isn't absorbed as well as iron from animal sources and because vitamin B_{12} is found almost exclusively in animal foods.

Eat foods rich in vitamin C at the same time that you eat whole grains, spinach, and legumes, in order to increase absorption of the iron they contain.

WHEN TO CALL THE DOCTOR

At the first sign of any of the following symptoms: weakness, unexplained fatigue, shortness of breath. That's because anemia can mask a more serious disease.

If you drink coffee or tea, do so between meals rather than with meals, because the caffeine in these beverages reduces iron absorption.

Super Supplements

Though most people can get adequate amounts of iron, vitamin B_{12}, and folic acid through their diet, experts believe that people who are at highest risk for nutrient deficiency anemias can benefit from taking supplements. If you are at higher-than-usual risk for a deficiency of iron, vitamin B_{12}, or folic acid, discuss it with your doctor, take a good look at your diet, and follow these recommendations.

- **Take it on empty.** The iron you absorb from supplements can be decreased by as much as 50 percent if you eat food with your supplement. Absorption is best when iron is taken on an empty stomach and washed down with juice or water.

- **Don't overload.** The government has done extensive testing on how much of a nutrient is adequate for a healthy diet. Overdoing the amounts can be harmful instead of beneficial. For example, taking too much folic acid may mask symptoms of pernicious anemia. Follow the Recommended Daily Allowances (RDAs) guideline.

- **Be a label reader.** Be cautious when choosing a supplement, and be sure that it meets your unique needs. Some vitamin supplements don't contain any folic acid at all. And some may contain large amounts of nutrients that you don't need, which can be not only a waste of money but, depending on the nutrients, also harmful to your health. In addition, be sure to check the expiration date on the bottle; you don't want to buy a 500-count bottle of a once-a-day supplement that expires in six months!

ATHLETE'S FOOT

Athlete's foot itches, burns, and is downright ugly to look at. But it's not a condition unique to athletes. Blame the misnomer on the ad man who gave it its name in the 1930s. In fact, athlete's foot, or *tinea pedis,* is the most common fungal infection of the skin. This fungus loves moist places, especially the soft, warm, damp skin between the toes. Certainly the athlete's locker room environment, with its steamy showers, is a good place for the fungus to thrive. But *tinea pedis* is actually present on most people's skin all the time, just waiting for the right opportunity to develop into an infection.

Who Gets It?

So what causes athlete's foot to rear its ugly little fungal head? Skin that's irritated, weakened, or continuously moist is primed for an athlete's foot infection. And certain medications, including antibiotics, corticosteroids, birth control pills, and drugs that suppress immune function, can make you more susceptible. People who are obese and those who have diabetes mellitus or a weakened immune system, such as those with AIDS, also are at increased risk. And some people may be genetically predisposed to developing athlete's foot.

Anyone can get athlete's foot—and most people will at some time in their lives. Teenage and adult males, though, are the most susceptible. They're at the top of the fungus-footed list. So who's at the bottom? The following are those who are least likely to succumb:

- People who spend a lot of time barefoot
- Women
- Children under the age of 12

Signs and Symptoms

Just because you're not in the high risk category doesn't mean you're safe. Here's how you can tell whether you have an athlete's foot infection:

- Itching, scaling, red skin
- Red, cracking, peeling skin between the toes
- Dry, flaking skin
- Blisters
- Unpleasant and unusual foot odor

Keep It from Spreading

In extreme cases, the fungus that causes athlete's foot can spread to other moist areas of the body, such as the groin and even the armpits. So take precautions when coming into contact with that athlete's foot. Be sure to wash your hands with soap and water after contact. Keep your linens and towels clean, and never wear the same pair of socks twice without first washing them. You can also spread athlete's foot with contaminated sheets, towels, and clothing.

There are any number of anti-fungal creams on the market that can rid you of your foot fungus. They're costly, and you may have to buy several tubes or cans before the problem is cleared. So before you trudge off to the pharmacy on those poor, itchy feet, try some of the following kitchen concoctions.

GARLIC RECIPE

Crush 1 clove garlic and mix with a few drops of olive oil to make a paste. Apply to the nail and leave on for 15 to 30 minutes, then clean off in warm, soapy water. Dry feet thoroughly. Repeat daily. Because the fungus can return, you may wish to continue this treatment for several weeks after it has disappeared just to ward off another fungal visit.

From the Cupboard

Baking soda. Sprinkle baking soda directly into your shoes to help absorb moisture.

Cornstarch. Rub cornstarch, which absorbs moisture, on your feet. Very lightly browned cornstarch is even better because any moisture content already contained in the corn-starch is removed, allowing for better absorption. To brown, sprinkle cornstarch on a pie plate and bake at 325°F for just a few minutes, until it looks brownish. Then dab some on your feet and toes.

Garlic. Eat some garlic, as it has anti-fungal properties. You can also swab the affected area with garlic juice or oregano oil twice a day.

Immune-boosting foods.

Salt. Soak your infected foot in warm salt water, using 1 teaspoon salt for each cup of water, for ten minutes. Dry your foot thoroughly, then dab some baking soda between your toes.

Tea. The tannic acid in tea is soothing, helps to dry the foot, and helps kill the fungus. Make a foot soak by putting 6 black tea bags in 1 quart warm water.

Vinegar. Soak your feet in 1 cup vinegar to 2 quarts water for 15 to 30 minutes every night. Or make a solution of 1 cup vinegar to 1 cup water, and apply it directly to the affected areas with a cotton ball. If the infection is severe and the skin is raw, the solution will sting. Make sure your feet are completely dry before putting on your socks or slippers.

Cider vinegar can also be used as a remedy. Mix equal parts apple cider (or regular) vinegar and ethyl alcohol. Dab on the affected areas.

AVOID THIS HOUSEHOLD REMEDY

One of the oldest folk remedies for athlete's foot is to soak your tootsies in diluted bleach water. The theory was that the bleach solution would dry out the skin and kill the infection. And it will do that. But the chlorine in the bleach is a harsh chemical, and it can cause skin damage while not necessarily killing the fungus. Be cautious about using chemicals and solvents such as bleach and alcohol. They may do more harm than good, despite the fact that many natural remedy practitioners still swear by the bleach treatment.

From the Refrigerator

Immune-boosting Foods. Low immunity can make you more susceptible to a fungal infection, so include some of these immune-boosting foods in your diet: broccoli, red meats, scallions, garlic, sweet potatoes, whole-grain breads, sunflower seeds, onions, and rice.

Lemon. This remedy will help you in the sweaty feet-odor department. Squeeze the juice from a lemon and mix it with 2 ounces water. Rinse your feet with the lemon water.

Yogurt. One of the greatest of all fungus-fighting foods in your fridge is yogurt that contains acidophilus. It doesn't matter what the flavor is as long as the yogurt contains the active bacteria (check the label; it will tell you). Acidophilus helps control vaginal and oral yeast, but it may give other fungi a pretty good fight, too. And if nothing else, it tastes good and is good for you, too!

From the Spice Rack

Cinnamon. A good soak in a cinnamon tea foot bath will help slow down the fungus. Boil 8 to 10 broken cinnamon sticks in 4 cups water, then simmer for five minutes. Let steep for another 45 minutes. Soak your feet for 15 to 30 minutes. Repeat daily as needed.

More Do's and Don'ts

- Don't wear tight-fitting or watertight shoes. Skip shoes made of plastic and rubber, too. The best shoe choices are those made of natural materials that "breathe," such as leather.

- Don't share or swap shoes with anybody. If you find yourself with a pair of someone else's vintage shoes, treat them with antifungal powder before you put them on.

- Wear sandals or thongs on your feet in fungus-harboring public places such as beach showers and locker rooms; don't go barefoot.

- Set your shoes outside to air on a warm, sunny day. This will help dry

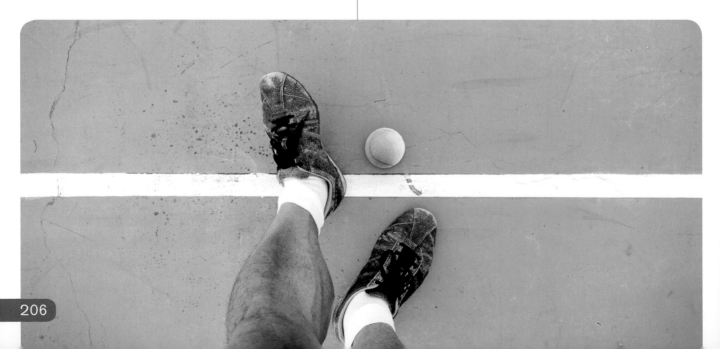

them out and kill the fungus. Alternate shoes every day. Wear one pair while you dry out the other.

- When selecting socks, try both natural and synthetic fabrics to see which keep your sweaty feet the driest. You may wish to try synthetic sock liners to absorb the moisture and keep it away from your skin.

- Give your socks a double washing in extra hot water to kill the fungal spores.

- Make sure to dry thoroughly between your toes after bathing. That's where athlete's foot usually starts.

WHEN TO CALL THE DOCTOR

- If the infections gets worse no matter what you do
- If one or both feet swell
- If you see pus in the cracks
- If the fungus spreads to your hands or elsewhere
- If you see an obvious change in color in your toenails, especially the nail of your big toe
- If you develop pain in the feet along with angry-looking inflammation, general malaise, fever, or chills. Your athlete's foot could be turning into a much more serious condition called cellulitis, which MUST be treated by a physician immediately.

When you're not in a wet environment, go barefooted as often as you can. This will get your foot outside the moist shoe environment where fungus loves to lurk. This is best done indoors, however, where you are less likely to cut, scrape, or otherwise injure your feet.

BRONCHITIS

That nasty cold has been hanging on much longer than it should, and day by day it seems to be getting worse. Your chest hurts, you gurgle when you breathe, and you're coughing so much yellow, green, or gray mucus that your throat is raw. These symptoms are letting you know that your cold has probably turned into a respiratory infection called bronchitis, an inflammation of the little branches and tubes of your windpipe that also makes them swell. No wonder breathing has become such a chore. Your air passages are too puffy to carry air very easily.

Acute bronchitis can include these other symptoms, too:

- Wheezing

- Shortness of breath

- Fever or chills

- General aches and pains

- Upper chest pain

Bronchitis is not contagious since it's a secondary infection that develops when your immune system is weakened by a cold or the flu. Some people are prone to developing it, some are not. Those at the top of the risk list have respiratory problems already, such as asthma, allergies, and emphysema. People who have a weakened immune system also are more prone to bronchitis. But anyone can develop it, and most people do at one time or another.

Under most circumstances, bronchitis will go away on its own once the primary infection is cured. But in those few days when you have it, it can sure be miserable. Here are a few tips that can relieve some of the symptoms.

ALMOND CREAM RECIPE

- 4 ounces whole almonds

- $\frac{1}{4}$ teaspoon pure vanilla extract (increase to $\frac{1}{2}$ if you're using imitation)

- honey

- cinnamon (optional)

Blanch almonds by covering with 1 / 2 cup plus 2 tablespoons water, and bring to a boil. Remove the skins, then puree in the blender with the water in which they cooked. Add vanilla. Add a pinch of cinnamon (optional). Sweeten to taste with a little honey.

From the Cupboard

Almonds. These little cure-all nuts have loads of vitamins and nutrients, and they are known to help everything from mental acuity to sexual vitality. Rich in potassium, calcium, and magnesium, almonds are especially known for their healing powers in respiratory illness. So when you're down with bronchitis, eat them in any form, except candy-coated or chocolate-covered. How about a little almond cream to drizzle over your oatmeal in the morning? Or sliver some almonds and garnish your veggies. They're good in a citrus fruit salad for a little added crunch or rubbed in a little honey, coated with cinnamon, and roasted in a 325°F oven for 10 to 25 minutes.

Coffee. The xanthine derivatives in coffee are good bronchodilators. To cut down on mucus problems, add 1 teaspoon apple cider vinegar and 2 drops peppermint oil to a cup of black coffee, either instant or brewed. Drink 1 cup in the morning and evening.

Honey. To relieve the cough that comes from bronchitis, slice an onion into a bowl, then cover with honey. Allow to stand overnight, then remove the onion. Take 1 teaspoon of the honey four times a day.

Salt. Make a saltwater gargle by mixing 1 teaspoon salt into a glass of warm water. The gargle is soothing, and it can cut down on mucus that's difficult to clear out of the throat. Just be sure not to use more salt, as it can burn your throat, or less salt, as it will be ineffective.

From the Refrigerator

Horseradish. The irritating allyl isothiocyanates (mustard derivatives) in horseradish open up the sinuses. Be careful not to use horseradish if you're having stomach problems, though, because it's too potent. Eat it straight, on a salad, or atop meat. Fresh horseradish is the best choice, but commercial products will work, too. Make sure it's straight horseradish, though. Sandwich spreads with horseradish won't work.

Lemons. These help rid the respiratory system of bacteria and mucus. Make a cup of lemon tea by grating 1 teaspoon lemon rind and adding it to 1 cup of boiling water. Steep for five minutes. Or, you can boil a lemon wedge. Strain into a cup and drink. For a sore throat that comes from coughing, add 1 teaspoon lemon juice to 1 cup warm water and gargle. This helps bring up phlegm.

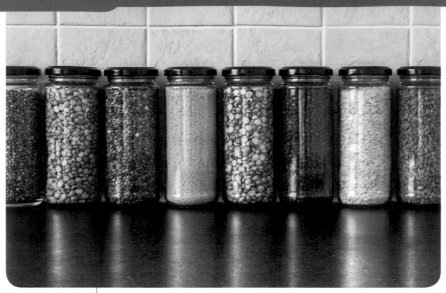

Onions. These are expectorants and help the flow of mucus. Use raw, cooked, baked, in soups and stews, as seasoning, or any which way you like them.

From the Sink

Water. Lots and lots of it. The more you drink, the more your mucus will liquify. This makes it easier to cough out. You can also use water for a steam treatment. Fill the sink with hot water, bend down to it, cover your head with a towel, and breathe in the steam. Add a few drops of eucalyptus, peppermint, or rosemary oil if you have one of them. These help clear and soothe the respiratory passages.

From the Spice Rack

Aniseed. Here's a bronchitis cough reliever that's also said to bring on breast milk and relieve heartburn. Boil 1 quart water, then add 7 teaspoons aniseed. Simmer until the water is half gone, strain the seeds, and add 4 teaspoons each of honey and glycerine (glycerine is available at the drugstore). Take 2 teaspoons every few hours.

Bay leaf. Ancient Romans and Greeks loved bay leaves. They believed that this simple herb was the source of happiness, clairvoyance, and artistic inspiration. Whatever the case, it does act as an expectorant and is best taken in tea. To make the tea, tear a leaf (fresh or dried) and steep in 1 cup boiling water. *Warning!* Bay leaf tea should not be used during pregnancy, as it may bring on menstruation. Another bronchitis remedy with bay leaf is to soak some leaves in hot water and apply as a poultice to the chest. Cover with a kitchen towel. As it cools, rewarm.

Ginger. This is a potent expectorant that works well in tea. Steep $\frac{1}{2}$ teaspoon ginger, a pinch of ground cloves, and a pinch of cinnamon in 1 cup boiling water.

Mustard. The warmth of an old-fashioned mustard plaster relieves symptoms of many respiratory ailments, including bronchitis. Take 1 tablespoon dry mustard and mix with 4 tablespoons flour. Stir in enough warm water to make a runny paste. Oil the chest with vegetable shortening or olive oil, then spread the mustard mix on a piece of cloth—muslin, gauze, a kitchen washcloth—and cover with an identical piece. Apply to the chest. Keep in place until cool, but check every few minutes to make sure it doesn't burn the skin. Remove the plaster if it causes discomfort or burning.

Savory. This potent, peppery herb is said to rid the lungs of mucus. Use it as a tea by adding $\frac{1}{2}$ teaspoon savory to 1 cup boiling water. Drink only once a day.

Thyme. This herb helps rid the body of mucus, strengthens the lungs to fight off infection, and acts as a shield against bacteria. Use it dried

---

BRONCHITIS-FRIENDLY FOODS

These won't cure, but studies indicate that foods rich in these nutrients may protect against another bout of bronchitis. The more vegetables you eat, the more protection you have.

Beta-Carotene: carrots, apricots, sweet potatoes, mangoes, green veggies

Vitamin E: green leafy veggies, avocados, whole-grain cereal

Vitamin A: mackerel, anchovies, canned red salmon, whole milk, cheese, egg yolks

Omega-3 fatty acids: herring, kippers, mackerel, salmon, sardines, trout, fresh tuna, crab

as a seasoning or make a tea by adding $\frac{1}{4}$ to $\frac{1}{2}$ teaspoon thyme (it's a very strong herb, so you don't need much) to 1 cup boiling water. Steep for 5 minutes and sweeten with honey. If you have thyme oil on hand, dilute it (2 parts olive or corn oil to 1 part thyme oil) and rub on the chest to cure congestion.

From the Stove

Humidity. You don't need a humidifier to get moisture into your lungs. Simmer a pot of water on the stove to send some steam into the atmosphere, which will kill germs and viruses. Or better yet, use a tea kettle: It's designed to shoot out that warm, moist air. And if you have a few drops of peppermint or eucalyptus oil to add, these can relieve congestion and be quite soothing.

Mucus-Makers to Avoid

When you're congested, there are a few simple foods that should be avoided because they produce more mucus.

WHEN TO CALL THE DOCTOR

- If symptoms last more than three to four days
- If your bronchitis keeps returning
- If the person with bronchitis is an infant or an older adult. Complications in these people can become very serious or even deadly.
- If you have a lot of greenish mucus. You may need antibiotics.
- If you have lung or heart disease, or any other debilitating chronic illness or immune problem
- If you cough up blood. Tiny bright red specks normally come from irritation to the airways, so a few specks of blood can be normal. Coughing up larger amounts or blood that is dried and brownish may require treatment.
- If your temperature lingers at 102°F for a couple of days

Here's the list:

- Dairy foods
- Sugary products, including carbonated and noncarbonated soft drinks; sugar-coated cereal; sugary throat lozenges
- Refined cereals, bread, pasta
- Fried and fatty foods
- Red meat, including pork

Here's a handy avoidance reminder: When you're congested, skip the white stuff—milk, flour, sugar.

More Do's and Don'ts

- Rest up. Then rest some more. Since bronchitis is usually the second half of a double-illness whammy, your body needs all the rest it can get to build up its strength.

- Don't take a cough suppressant unless your doctor prescribes it. Coughing is your body's way of getting rid of mucus. Mucus buildup can lead to serious respiratory complications such as pneumonia, so when you're congested, that cough is your friend!

- Stay out of harm's way. With bronchitis you're at risk for picking up another infection. Avoid crowds, children with colds, smoky rooms, and contact with anyone who has a cold or flu. Wear gloves or a mask if you have to.

- Wash your hands often: after using a phone, handling a contaminated tissue, or shaking hands with someone who may have a cold or a virus.

- Pamper yourself. Go to bed, read a book, listen to music, watch an old movie. Don't be tempted to go about business as usual just because bronchitis isn't usually contagious or serious.

COLDS

Every year Americans will suffer through more than one billion colds. That's one billion runny noses, coughs, sneezes, aches, and sore throats. Colds make such frequent appearances that the infection has come to be known as the "common cold."

Small children are the most likely to catch a cold: Most kids will have six to ten colds a year. That's because their young immune systems combined with the germy confines of school and day-care situations make them prime targets for the virus. The upside of having so many colds as a child is that you develop immunities to some of the 200 viruses that cause colds. As a result, adults get an average of only two to four colds a year. By the time most people reach age 60, they're down to about one cold per year. Women, however, especially women between 20 and 30 years old, get more colds than men.

How Do Colds Beat a Path to Your Door?

Viruses are like the bully that torments all the kids on the playground. After entering the mucous layer of your nose and throat, the cold virus strong-arms your cells until they let the virus take over, forcing the cells to produce thousands of new virus particles.

But the virus is not the reason your throat begins throbbing and your nose starts flowing like Niagara Falls. Your immune system is responsible for that. As the virus begins replicating, the body gets the message that it's time to go into battle. The little soldiers of the body, the white blood cells, run to the body's rescue. One of the weapons the white blood cells use in their virus war are immune system chemicals called kinins. During the battle the kinins tell the body to go into defensive mode. So that runny nose is really your body fighting back against the cursed virus. That should make you feel a little better while you lie on the couch surrounded by tissues.

Because there are so many viruses that cause colds, the exact virus that you contracted is not easily pinned down. The most likely culprit in most colds is a rhinovirus (rhino is a Greek word meaning "nose"). There are over 110 specific rhinoviruses, and they are behind 30 to 35 percent of most colds. The second most common reason for that aching head is a coronavirus. These are especially common in adults. An unknown viral assailant causes 30 to 50 percent of colds, and about 10 to 15 percent of colds are caused by a virus that will probably lead to something more serious, such as the flu.

How Colds Are Spread

The cold virus can take many routes to its ultimate destination—your cells. Most people are contagious a day before and two to four days after their symptoms start. There are typically three ways a cold virus is spread:

- Touching someone who has the virus on them. The virus can live for three hours on skin.
- Touching something that contains

YOU CAN'T CATCH A COLD FROM COLD

Cold weather may make you uncomfortable, but it doesn't make you more susceptible to getting a cold. There are two reasons colds tend to make more of an impact in cold weather. Number one, most people are indoors a lot more in the winter, so you've got a lot more opportunities to share the wealth of cold viruses. And number two, the heat in your house dries out the air, and cold viruses like it warm and dry. So if you throw a little wintertime soiree in your well-heated home, you've got the ideal climate for a cold virus. Scientists have done numerous tests in which they've exposed people to the cold virus in 86°F and 40°F temperatures, and much to the participants' chagrin, both groups ended up with a cold.

the virus. Cold viruses can live three hours on objects.

- Inhaling the virus through airborne transmission. It may sound implausible, but if someone sitting next to you sneezes while you are inhaling, voilà! It's likely you'll get a cold.

One study found that kids tend to get colds from more direct contact while adults tend to get colds from airborne viruses (moms of young children can expect to get colds both ways). Research has also found that emotional stress, allergies that affect the nasal passages or throat, and menstrual cycles may make you more susceptible to catching a cold.

Where's the Cold Vaccine?

Good question! One of the main reasons we don't yet have a vaccine for the cold is that they're just too hard to pin down. Viruses live inside cells, which means they are protected from most medicines in the bloodstream. So even if you took an antiviral drug, chances are your body wouldn't allow it to penetrate the cells. Another reason viruses are so difficult to kill is that they don't grow well in a laboratory setting. Their ultimate playground is a cool, dry place, just like the inside of your nose.

Don't give up hope, though. Researchers are still on the job. Scientists have discovered the receptor sites that the rhinovirus attaches to when it invades a cell. They tested an antibody that blocked these receptor sites and helped slow down the time the virus actually took to develop into a cold. It also reduced the severity of its symptoms.

While colds are here to stay for now, you don't have to be totally at their mercy. Thankfully, there are some things you can do to fend off the germs that cause colds, as well as techniques to ease your symptoms once you're sick.

How to Win the Cold War

Washing your hands is the most effective way to keep a cold at bay as well as to keep one from spreading. Antibacterial soaps don't necessarily do any more good than regular soap, and some researchers believe the prevalence of antibacterial products is contributing to the increase in resistant bacteria strains. Experts suggest washing your hands for at least 15 seconds—long enough to say the alphabet. So next time you're scrubbing, just say those ABCs.

Always sneeze or cough into a tissue and throw it away immediately. Sounds like a no-brainer, but how many tissues

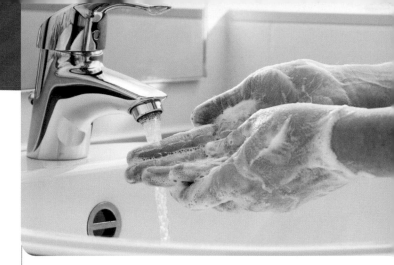

have you just left sitting around the house?

Clean any potentially virus-carrying surface of your home with a heavy-duty cleanser or disinfectant.

Try not to hang around people who have colds, and try to limit your exposure to others if you have a cold.

Cures from the Cupboard

Chicken soup. Science actually backs up what your mom knew all along—chicken soup does help a cold. Scientists believe it's the fumes in the soup that release the mucus in your nose and help your body better fight against its viral invaders. Chicken soup also contains cysteines, which are good at thinning mucus. And the soup provides easily absorbed nutrients.

Corn syrup. You can make a sugar-water gargle to ease your throat. Use 1 tablespoon syrup per 8 ounces warm water, mix together, and gargle.

Honey. Make your own cough syrup by mixing together $\frac{1}{4}$ cup honey and $\frac{1}{4}$ cup apple cider vinegar. Pour the mixture into a jar or bottle and seal tightly. Shake well before using. Take 1 tablespoon every four hours.

Salt. Make your own saline drops by adding $\frac{1}{4}$ teaspoon salt to 8 ounces water. You can also make a saltwater gargle for your sore throat with the same ratio of salt to water. Salt is an astringent and helps relieve a painful throat.

Sesame Oil. Although doctors typically recommend saline nose drops during the winter to keep nasal passages moist, one study compared saline drops to sesame oil. People who used sesame oil had an 80 percent improvement in their nasal dryness while people who used traditional saline drops had a 30 percent improvement. While it may not be a good idea to shoot sesame oil up your nose (it could get into the lungs), try rubbing a drop around the inside of your nostrils.

Tea. A cup of hot tea with honey does the same trick as chicken soup; it loosens up your nasal passages and makes that stuffy nose feel better. Folk healers have known this secret for centuries. They often suggest drinking tea with spices and herbs that contain aromatic oils with antiviral properties. Try tea with elder, ginger, yarrow, mint, thyme, horsemint, bee balm, lemon balm, catnip, garlic, onions, or mustard.

From the Refrigerator

Peppers. Hot and spicy foods are notorious for making your nose run and your eyes water. The hot stuff in peppers is called capsaicin and is pharmacologically similar to guaifenesin, an expectorant found in some over-the-counter cough syrups. This similarity leads some experts to believe that eating hot foods can clear up mucus and ease that stuffy nose.

Yogurt. One study found that participants who ate ¾ cup yogurt a day before and during cold season had 25 percent fewer colds. But you've got to start early and maintain your yogurt eating throughout the peak cold season.

From the Supplement Shelf

Vitamin C. Vitamin C won't prevent a cold, but research shows that it can help reduce the length and severity of symptoms. But to reap the benefits, you've got

---

A HEALING HERB

Echinacea's immune-stimulating properties have been proved in European tests. A favorite in folk medicine for centuries, echinacea is used in contemporary herbal treatments in Britain, Australia, and the United States. In Germany, where herbs are prescribed just like pharmaceutical medicines, this handy herb is prescribed for colds. German clinical tests have shown that echinacea can help decrease cold symptoms. For the best results, take echinacea at the onset of cold symptoms—but not for longer than two weeks.

to take a lot of "C." The RDA for men and women 15 and older is 60 mg, but studies show that you'd need to take upward of 1,000 mg to 3,000 mg to get the cold-symptom-sparing rewards of vitamin C. For the short term, experts believe that wouldn't be harmful, but taking too much vitamin C for too long can cause severe diarrhea. Before loading up on vitamin C, check with your doctor.

Zinc. Studies have found that zinc may help immune cells fight a cold and may ease cold symptoms. The most effective zinc lozenges are those that contain 15 to 25 mg of zinc gluconate or zinc gluconate-glycine per lozenge. You

WHEN TO CALL THE DOCTOR

Colds generally have to run their course, typically about 2 to 14 days. In rare cases, they can lead to a more serious infection. Call your doctor if you have

- High fever
- Severe pain in the chest, ears, head, or stomach
- Enlarged lymph nodes (glands in the neck)
- A fever, sore throat, or severe runny nose that doesn't get any better in a week
- A headache and stiff neck but no other symptoms (could be meningitis)
- A headache and sore throat but no other symptoms (could be strep throat)
- Typical cold symptoms and pain across your nose and face that sticks around (could be a sinus infection)
- Lessening cold symptoms but then the sudden onset of fever (could be pneumonia)

can get the most out of your zinc lozenges if you start using them at the first sign of a cold and continue taking them for several days.

More Do's and Don'ts

- Don't fix yourself a hot toddy; they don't work. Alcohol can make you more stuffy. Best to avoid it while you've got a cold.

- Don't smoke. Smokers tend to have longer colds, and they're more likely to end up with complications, such as bronchitis.

- Don't take antibiotics. Antibiotics don't fight viral infections, so they

- aren't effective against colds. And taking too many antibiotics can build up immunity, so when you truly need an antibiotic your body will be resistant to its healing properties.

- Keep your chin up. Just as emotional stress can wear your immune system down, having a positive attitude can help you win the war against your cold.

Watch the Medicines

During cold season, you'll find tons of commercials for over-the-counter cold remedies. They may make you feel better temporarily, but they may also make your cold stick around longer. That runny nose and cough are your body's way of getting rid of all the virus. But if you desperately need some relief, avoid multi-symptom cold medicines. Stick with medicines that treat your specific symptom, such as a stuffy nose or a dry cough.

DIARRHEA

It's got all kinds of colorful nicknames, including "Greased Lightning," "Turkey Trots," and "Montezuma's Revenge." You may have even heard your 11-year-old singing a catchy little ditty about it. But just saying the word diarrhea gets a reaction from most people—they either giggle or turn pale. Diarrhea is probably one of the most unpleasant problems that plagues us. And it's a common malady. Americans usually suffer from diarrhea a couple times a year. For most adults, diarrhea isn't serious. And it does give you a chance to ponder some redecorating ideas for the bathroom.

The Rundown on Diarrhea

On a typical day, you eat a hoagie and drink an iced tea and your meal makes its way through the digestive system without any problems. By the time it reaches the intestines, your food is mostly fluid with bits of solid material. The intestines reabsorb most of the fluid, and the solid stuff is excreted in the usual fashion. But when you've got diarrhea, something blocks the intestine's ability to absorb fluid. You've got loads of watery fluids mixed in with your stool, and you get that "gotta go" feeling.

There are essentially two types of diarrhea: acute and chronic. Thankfully, the vast majority of diarrhea is acute, or short term. This type of diarrhea keeps you on the toilet for a couple of days but doesn't stick around long. Acute diarrhea is also known as non-inflammatory diarrhea. Its symptoms are what most people associate with the condition: watery, frequent stools accompanied by stomach cramps, gas, and nausea.

Acute diarrhea usually has a bacterial or viral culprit. Gastroenteritis, mistakenly called the "stomach flu," is one of the most common infections that cause diarrhea. Gastroenteritis can be caused by many different viruses. Eating or drinking foods contaminated with bacteria can also cause diarrhea. Other causes of acute diarrhea are lactose intolerance, sweeteners such as sorbitol, over-the-counter antacids that contain magnesium, too much vitamin C, and some antibiotics.

If you have chronic, or long-term, diarrhea that comes on suddenly and stays for weeks, you may have a more serious condition such as irritable bowel syndrome or a severe food allergy.

Dehydration Dangers

With any kind of diarrhea you lose a lot of fluids. One of the quickest ways you can end up going from the bathroom to the emergency room is to take a pass on liquids while you're sick. Fluids not only keep things running smoothly in your body, they also keep electrolyte levels balanced. Electrolytes are sodium, potassium, and chloride salts that your body needs for proper organ function. An electrolyte imbalance can cause your heart to beat irregularly, causing life-threatening problems. Though drinking or eating anything while you're running back and forth to the bathroom might sound grotesque, it will help make you more comfortable and get you back on your feet more quickly.

Though experts don't see eye to eye on what fluids are best during a bout with diarrhea, they do agree that getting two to three quarts of fluid a day is a good idea. When you drink, it's easier on the tummy if you sip instead of gulp (who has the energy for gulping?) and if you drink cool, not cold or hot, fluids. Here are some tried-and-true fluids that should get you through the rough days.

- Decaffeinated tea with a little sugar
- Sports drinks
- Commercially available electrolyte replacement drinks for children
- Bouillon
- Chicken broth
- Orange juice

Though it may not sound logical to put diarrhea and food in the same sentence, if you don't put something in your body while you're enduring tummy troubles, you might end up getting sicker. There are loads of good things from the kitchen that will ease your grumbling stomach, and there are a few things that will prevent those diarrhea-causing agents from coming back for a return engagement.

From the Cupboard

Blueberries. Blueberry root is a long-time folk remedy for diarrhea. In Sweden, doctors prescribe a soup made with dried blueberries for tummy problems. Blueberries are rich in anthocyanosides, which have antioxidant and antibacterial properties, as well as tannins, which combat diarrhea.

Chamomile tea. Chamomile is good for treating intestinal inflammation, and it has antispasmodic properties as well. You can brew yourself a cup of chamomile tea from packaged tea bags, or you can buy chamomile flowers and steep 1 teaspoon of them and 1 teaspoon of peppermint leaves in a cup of boiling water for fifteen minutes. Drink 3 cups a day.

Cooked cereals. Starchy foods, such as precooked rice or tapioca cereals, can help ease your tummy. Prepare the cereal according to the directions on the box, making it as thick as you can stomach it. Just avoid adding too much sugar or salt, as these can aggravate diarrhea. It's probably a good idea to avoid oatmeal since it's high in fiber and your intestines can't tolerate the added bulk during a bout with diarrhea.

Potatoes. This is another starchy food that can help restore nutrients and comfort your stomach. But eating French fries won't help. Fried foods tend to aggravate an aching tummy. Other root vegetables such as carrots (cooked, of course) are also easy on an upset stom-ach, and they are happily loaded with nutrients.

Rice. Cooked white rice is another starchy food that can be handled by someone recovering from diarrhea.

Sugar. To make your own fluid replacement, mix 4 teaspoons sugar and $\frac{1}{2}$ teaspoon salt with 1 quart water. Mixing electrolytes (such as salt) with a form of glucose (sugar) helps the body to better absorb the nutrients.

From the Fruit Basket

Banana. Long known as a soother for tummy trouble, this potassium-rich fruit can restore nutrients and is easy to digest.

WHEN TO CALL THE DOCTOR

Most diarrhea has to run its course. However, diarrhea can be a sign of a more serious problem. If you're concerned, here are some symptoms that warrant a trip to the emergency room or a call to your family physician.

- Your diarrhea symptoms last more than 48 hours
- You have severe stomach cramps
- You have blood or pus in your stool
- You start showing any signs of severe dehydration such as dizziness when you stand, urinating less frequently or in very small amounts, dark yellow urine, increased thirst, and dry skin
- You have fever or chills

Orange peel. Orange peel tea is a folk remedy that is believed to aid in digestion. Place a chopped orange peel (preferably from an organic orange, as peels otherwise may contain pesticides and dyes) into a pot and cover with 1 pint boiling water. Let it stand until the water is cooled. You can sweeten it with sugar or honey.

From the Refrigerator

Yogurt. Look for yogurt with live cultures. These "cultures" are friendly bacteria that can go in and line your intestines, providing you protection from the bad guys. If you've already got diarrhea, yogurt can help produce lactic acid

MILK'S NOT ALWAYS GOOD FOR YOU

Between 70 and 90 percent of Asian, African-American, Native American, and Mediterranean adults lack the enzyme lactase, which is responsible for digesting lactose, a sugar found in milk. Lactose intolerance is the most common reason for chronic diarrhea.

in your intestines, which can kill off the nasty bacteria and get you feeling better, faster.

From the Spice Rack

Fenugreek seeds. Science has given the nod to this folk remedy. But this one is for adults only. Mix ½ teaspoon fenugreek seeds with water and drink up.

More Do's and Dont's

- To ease stomach pain, try resting with a heating pad on your belly.

- Don't take antidiarrheal medications at the onset of your illness. Let your body rid itself of whatever's causing the problem first.

- Wash your hands thoroughly before preparing food. You don't want to pass your illness to everyone in the household.

Foods to Avoid

Caffeine. It stimulates the nervous system, including the intestines.

Sweeteners such as sorbitol, xylitol, and mannitol. These are mostly found in fruit juices, such as apple juice, and sugarless candy.

Milk and cheese. The intestines work extra hard to digest the enzymes in these dairy products. While your body is down for the count, and even a few days after you're better, you might want to avoid dairy of any kind except for yogurt.

Fiber. Now is not the time to bulk up. Fiber is simply too hard for an aching tummy to digest.

Sugar: Some sugar is good during a case of diarrhea—it can help you absorb electrolytes needed for rehydration—but too much can make things worse.

Babies and Seniors Need Special Care

Because they have a smaller blood volume than adults, babies can dehydrate in minutes and children can dehydrate in hours. And many elderly people have slower circulatory systems because of hardening of the arteries and thus simply can't afford to be low on fluids. Members of these groups need special care.

Call the doctor for babies as soon as they have a loose stool. Though it may be hard to tell in a breast-fed baby, since their stools are already loose, if you have any question that it might be diarrhea, err on the side of caution. The same is true for seniors; call the doctor as soon as you have a loose bowel movement. Your diarrhea might be the side effect of a medication, such as an antibiotic, and it needs to be remedied without delay.

Call the doctor or head to the emergency room if your baby:

- has fewer wet diapers
- has dark yellow urine
- has dry, pale skin that's cool to the touch
- has a dry tongue
- is not drooling
- is thirsty
- has a rapid pulse
- has sunken eyes

- cries but has no tears
- has a sunken fontanel (soft spot)

Avoiding Traveler's Diarrhea

The announcer said, "Congratulations, you've just won a five-day, four-night stay at a posh resort in the tropical paradise of your choice." Unfortunately, he didn't mention that paradise came with a bevy of food-borne parasites. Forty to sixty percent of Americans who travel abroad will end up with a case of traveler's diarrhea, usually within four to six days of arrival in a foreign country. It's most often caused by a bacteria, such as *E. coli,* that wanders into the intestines and beds down. Once you've got it, it can take hold with a vengeance and last for weeks.

You can avoid getting traveler's diarrhea by avoiding the bacteria that cause it. The best way to do that is to read up on potential bacterial invasions in your country of choice—see the Centers for Disease Control Web site www.cdc.gov to get a lowdown on your destination. And take these practical precautions.

- Make sure raw foods are cooked or boiled. Don't eat anything that appears rare. If you are eating fruit, make sure it has a peel.

- Take care of your own stuff. Peel your own fruit. Open your own bottle of water. The fruit on the buffet table may have been washed in contaminated water. That open bottle of water could be from the tap.

- Go back on the bottle. Drink only bottled water, preferably the bubbly kind. Carbonation seems to kill some bacteria. If you can't get bottled water, invest in a portable water filter.

- Don't drink the water. Don't drink tap water in any form—spritzed over vegetables, in the form of ice cubes, in a pitcher of lemonade, etc.

- Eat it hot. Only eat food that is hot to the touch, and eat as quickly as you can. Food that has cooled is a prime spot for nasty bacteria.

If you do get diarrhea and aren't careful to replace the fluid you're losing, you might be in danger of dehydrating. There are certain age-groups, such as children and the elderly, who are more in danger of dehydrating, and special care needs to be taken when they have diarrhea.

FLU (INFLUENZA)

Boo hoo if you've got the flu. Unlike the common cold, which causes a stuffy nose, sore throat, and sneezing, the flu is a viral infection that strikes the entire body with a vengeance. The misery starts suddenly with chills and fever and spirals into more unpleasant symptoms that will take you out of commission: a sore throat, dry cough, stuffy or runny nose, headache, nausea, vomiting, severe muscle aches and pains, weakness, backache, and loss of appetite. Some people even experience pain and stiffness in the joints.

The worst of your symptoms will last about three to five days, but others, such as cough and fatigue, can linger for weeks. And a bout with the flu can deliver a double whammy if you develop a secondary infection, such as an ear or sinus infection or bronchitis. Even pneumonia can be a complication—and a potentially serious one—of influenza.

Flu viruses strike like clockwork in the United States. Every year they begin to show up in October and exit in April. Peak flu season takes place in December and January.

Flu is a highly contagious illness, spread by droplets from the respiratory tract of an infected person. These can be airborne, such as those released after a person coughs or sneezes, or they can be transferred via an infected person's hands. Taking a yearly flu shot can help you ward off infection, and these are particularly recommended for senior citizens, people with compromised immune systems, or people with asthma. They won't give you 100 percent protection, but they will significantly increase your chances of avoiding it.

If you do get the flu, there are kitchen remedies to help ease your suffering.

From the Cupboard

Broth. Canned broth, whether it's beef, chicken, or vegetable, will keep you hydrated and help liquefy any mucous secretions. Broth is easy to keep down, even when you have no appetite, and will provide at least some nutrients.

Honey. A hacking cough can keep you and every other household member up all night. Keep the peace with honey. Honey has long been used in traditional Chinese medicine for coughs. It's a simple enough recipe: Mix 1 tablespoon honey into 1 cup hot water, stir well, and enjoy. Honey acts as a natural expectorant, promoting the flow of mucus. Squeeze some lemon in if you want a little tartness.

MYTHS AND FACTS

Myth #1: The 24-hour flu. Fact: There is no such thing as a 24-hour flu, although we wish it were so. The sudden onslaught of vomiting, diarrhea, and a general feeling of malaise that is intense for a few hours, but subsides after 24 hours, is indeed caused by a viral agent, but not the one that causes influenza. The correct term should be "the 24-hour attack of gastroenteritis," which is an infection that affects the gastrointestinal tract.

Myth #2: Going outside without a hat or catching a chill causes the flu. Fact: Venturing outside ill-prepared for the elements may not be the brightest idea, but it doesn't directly cause the flu. Several scientific studies have shown that people exposed to cold temperatures for several hours fare no worse than those kept toasty warm. This myth grows from the observation that a severe chill is one of the first flu symptoms. Thus, people conclude that being chilled leads to the flu.

Mustard. Not to discredit dear old Grandma, but she didn't come up with the mustard plaster, although by the way she touts its virtues, you might believe so. Actually, this ancient remedy for the flu, chest colds, and bronchitis dates back to the ancient Romans, who early on understood the healing properties of mustard. Mustard is loaded with antimicrobial and anti-inflammatory properties, many of which can be inhaled through the vapors. Impress Grandma by making a mustard plaster with 1 tablespoon dry mustard and 2 to 4 tablespoons flour. Mix both with 1 egg white (optional) and warm water to form a paste. Next, find a clean handkerchief or square of muslin large enough to cover the upper chest. Smear the cloth the same way you'd smear mustard on a sandwich, then plop another cloth over it. Dab olive oil on the patient's skin and apply the mustard plaster to the upper chest. Check yourself or the patient every few minutes since mustard plaster can burn. Remove after a few minutes. Afterward, wash off any traces of mustard from the skin.

Tea. A cup of hot tea is just another way to take your fluids, which are so essential when you have the flu. Just be sure to choose decaffeinated varieties. Caffeine is a mild diuretic, which is counterproductive when you have the flu, and you certainly don't want to be awakened with the need to use the bathroom when you need your rest!

From the Refrigerator

Juice. Any flavor or kind will do. Just drink lots of juice both to keep yourself hydrated and to give yourself some extra vitamins.

Lemon. The lovely lemon may cause a puckered face if eaten raw, but in a hot beverage lemons will have you smiling. Hot lemonade has been used as a flu remedy since Roman times and is still highly regarded in the folk traditions of New England. Lemons, being highly acidic, help make mucous membranes distasteful to bacteria and viruses. Lemon oil, which gives the juice its fragrance, is like a wonder drug containing antibacterial, antiviral, antifungal, and anti-inflammatory constituents. The oil also acts as an expectorant. To make this flu-fighting fruit drink, place 1 chopped lemon—skin, pulp, and all—into 1 cup boiling water. While the lemon steeps for 5 minutes, inhale the steam. Strain, add honey (to taste), and enjoy. Drink hot lemonade three to four times a day throughout your illness.

From the Spice Rack

Pepper. Pepper is an irritant (try sniffling some), yet this annoying characteristic is a plus for those suffering from coughs with thick mucus. The irritating property of pepper stimulates circulation and the flow of mucus. Place 1 teaspoon black pepper into a cup and sweeten things up with the addition of 1 tablespoon honey. Fill with boiling water, let steep for 10 to 15 minutes, stir, and sip.

Thyme. It's time to try thyme when the mucous membranes are stuffed, the head aches, and the body is hot with fever. Wonderfully fragrant, thyme delights the senses (if you can smell when sick) and works as a powerful expectorant and antiseptic, thanks to its constituent oil, thymol. By cupping your hands around a mug of thyme tea and breathing in the steam, the thymol sets to work through your upper respiratory tract, loosening mucus and inhibiting bacteria from settling down to stay. Make thyme tea in a

snap by adding 1 teaspoon dried thyme leaves to 1 cup boiling water. Let steep for five minutes while inhaling the steam. Strain the tea, sweeten with honey (to taste), and slowly sip.

Herbal Remedies

You may not ordinarily keep these herbs in your kitchen, but it's a good idea to stock up on them before flu seasons starts. Then you can put together some soothing remedies for influenza symptoms.

Lemon balm. For adults who can't catch their zzz's while coping with the flu, lemon balm acts as a mild sedative. It also contains antiviral compounds to help disinfect mucous membranes. To make this relaxing potion, place 1 teaspoon dried lemon balm in 1 cup boiling water. Cover and let steep for ten minutes. Strain, sweeten with honey (to taste), and drink up to 4 cups a day. (Note: Lemon balm is also known as balm mint, bee balm, blue balm, garden balm, Melissa, and sweet balm.)

Peppermint. Running a fever of 102°F to 104°F is common with the flu. A way to cool your hot head, via sweating, is with a cup of peppermint tea. As an added bonus, peppermint contains menthol, which works as a decongestant to help unstuff sinuses. And peppermint has antispasmodic properties to help that hack. To make this fever fighter, place $\frac{1}{2}$ ounce peppermint leaves in a 1-quart jar of boiling water. Cover and let steep 20 minutes. Strain the liquid, add a cube of sugar if you'd like, and enjoy 2 to 3 cups a day.

Thyme and Peppermint. Variety is the spice of life! Combine thyme and peppermint to make an herbal steam broth that will deliver healing aromas to your aching nose and throat. Combine 1 $\frac{1}{2}$ quarts boiling water and 2 tablespoons each of dried thyme and peppermint in a large pot. Cover and steep for five minutes. Place the pot on a table and remove the lid. Lean in and cover both your head and the pot of steaming herbs with a large towel. Slowly breathe the herbal broth for 15 minutes. (*Warning:* Don't stick your nose too close to the broth or you'll risk a burn.)

WHEN TO CALL THE DOCTOR

- If flu symptoms are accompanied by a high fever that lasts more than three days
- If a cough persists, becomes worse, or is associated with chest pains and shortness of breath
- If the flu drags on and you don't get better
- If you have lung or heart disease, consult your physician at the first sign of flu. The elderly and the very young should also be taken to a doctor at the first sign of flu.

More Do's and Don'ts

- Get plenty of rest. Okay, you may not need to be told this, at least when the flu first hits. But rest is essential to allow your body to fight the virus. So indulge yourself, since you've got a good reason to rest.

- Drink lots of fluids. Water's good, as are teas, juice, and soups. Off-limits are coffee and soda pop, as they may contain caffeine and have no nutritional benefits whatsoever.

- If you have lots of aches and pains and just can't get comfortable, use an over-the-counter pain reliever. But don't give aspirin to anyone under age 18 because of the risk of Reye's syndrome, a potentially fatal illness that is linked with aspirin use and the flu in young people.

FOOD POISONING

The company's annual 4th of July barbecue started out a huge success. The ribs were superb. The potato salad was excellent. Even Helen's famous coleslaw got rave reviews. But about the time the sun went down, people started sprinting in all directions, and they weren't running in the three-legged race. Most of them were headed for the nearest bathroom. Food poisoning claims another round of victims.

The Centers for Disease Control and Prevention estimates that there will be about 76 million cases of food poisoning this year. It's an estimate because most cases of food poisoning go unreported, chalked up to the stomach flu or another bug. Even though the United States has strict guidelines when it comes to processing and handling food, there is always a risk of some food becoming contaminated. Ironically, though many cases of food poisoning do happen in restaurants, the most common place for foodborne illnesses to strike is your very own kitchen.

Bacteria's Bad Boys

There are somewhere around 100 bacteria that can cause food poisoning. But these are on "Most Wanted" list:

Campylobacter jejuni. A common cause of foodborne illness, this bacteria is found in raw and undercooked poultry and meat, unpasteurized milk, and untreated water. Cook food properly and clean hands and utensils to kill it.

Clostridium perfringens. Known as the "buffet germ," this bacteria grows fastest in casseroles, stews, and gravies that are held at low or room temperature. Make sure hot foods are kept hot and cold foods cold.

Escherichia coli (E. Coli) 0157:H7. This specific strain of E. coli can cause severe problems. Found mostly in raw or undercooked ground beef or unpasteurized milk, kill this bacteria by cooking food properly.

Salmonella. Found mostly in raw or undercooked meat, poultry, eggs, and fish, and in unpasteurized milk, salmonella is easy to get rid of. Cook foods thoroughly and drink only pasteurized milk.

Staphylococcus aureus. Staph bacteria is found on people (skin, nose, throat) but is spread through contaminated foods. It can't be killed by cooking; avoid this one by keeping hands and kitchen utensils clean.

Vibrio vulnificus. This bacteria is found in raw oysters and raw or undercooked mussels, clams, and whole scallops.

How Spoiled Food Makes You Feel

The symptoms you have after eating a pork chop laden with bad bacteria can range from mild (a few stomach cramps) to severe (you spend a couple of days camped out on the bathroom floor). Many people describe food poisoning as akin to being hit by a very large truck. The most common symptoms are diarrhea, stomach pain, cramping, nausea, and vomiting.

Because most of the symptoms of food poisoning are similar to those of other illnesses, such as a stomach virus, people aren't always sure food is the problem. If you think you've got food poisoning but aren't sure, take note: Most people get sick about 4 to 48 hours after eating the suspect food. And if you got sick, chances are everyone else who ate a contaminated chop will be sick, too.

Foiling Food Poisoning

You've had some potato salad that's been sitting in the sun too long. Your stomach starts to cramp, and you make your first trip to the bathroom. Now what? There's not really anything you can do to stop the symptoms of food poisoning once they start, and you shouldn't try. As awful as it is, the diarrhea and vomiting that happen when you contract a foodborne illness help your body get rid of the poison. Taking over-the-counter medications that halt the process can make you sicker. The best thing you can do is take care of yourself while you're sick. These kitchen remedies can at least make dealing with the symptoms more bearable and get you feeling better faster. There are also some things in your kitchen that will help prevent food poisoning from visiting your house.

From the Cupboard

Bleach. Scrubbing your counter with warm soapy water and bleach is one of your best defenses against bacteria that tend to hover on countertops. It's a good idea to clean your cutting boards in a bleach and water solution: Try soaking them in a mixture of 2 teaspoons bleach to 1 quart water. Let the boards air dry.

KEEPING BACTERIA AT BAY

Food that's very hot or very cold won't allow bacteria to grow. Here are the important numbers to know:

160°F: The food temperature at which you can begin saying "sayonara" to bacteria.

140°F: Foods cooked and held at this temperature won't be free of bacteria, but bacteria will not be able to spread.

125°F: At this temperature, bacteria can survive and a few will grow.

60°F: If risky food is left at this temperature for too long, bacteria will begin to take over.

40°F: The magic temperature at which potentially dangerous bacteria begin to grow.

32°F: Though most bacteria are halted at this temp, some bacteria will grow.

0°F: Bacteria don't die at this frigid temperature, but you can keep them from spreading.

Chicken soup. Once you start feeling a bit better, start your stomach out with bland foods. Chicken soup is tasty and easy to digest.

Sugar. Sugar helps your body hold onto fluid, and adding a spoonful of sugar to a glass of water or a cup of decaffeinated tea may be more palatable if you find sports drinks too sugary.

From the Fruit Bowl

Banana. As you spend more time embracing the porcelain throne, your body is losing essential elements like potassium. Losing these vital nutrients can make that I've-been-hit-by-a-truck feeling worse. Once you've come to a lull in the bathroom visitations, usually after the first 24 hours, try eating a banana. It's easy on your stomach and can make you feel a bit better.

From the Refrigerator

Sports drinks. Losing all that fluid means you're losing electrolytes (salts that keep your body functioning properly) and water. Replacing that fluid with a sports drink will help replace needed electrolytes, and the sugar in the drink will help your body better absorb the fluid it needs. If the sugar is too much for your tummy, tone the drink down by diluting it with water.

Water. You may not feel like having anything pass your lips, but you've got to stay hydrated, especially when you are losing fluids from both ends. Start off with a few sips of this easy-to-swallow liquid and work your way up to more substantial stuff.

More Do's and Don'ts

- Use a hot water bottle or a heating pad to ease your stomach cramps.

- Get lots of rest. Not that you'd feel like running a marathon or even attempting to go to the office, but take it easy at home. Stick to the bed or the couch, and let time do its magic.

- Don't start back on foods that are hard to digest. Give your stomach and your intestines time to recuperate. Stay away from spicy, smoked, fried, or salty foods. Stay away from raw vegetables or rich pastries or candies, and don't drink alcohol.

- Tell the health department about your woes. Telling your story may keep others from experiencing the same problems, especially if you experienced food poisoning after eating at a restaurant or other food establishment.

- Once you're sick, get someone else to go to the kitchen for you. You could be spreading more harmful bacteria and inviting others to share in your suffering.

- Wash your hands thoroughly before preparing food. You don't want to be like Typhoid Mary and pass your illness to everyone in the household.

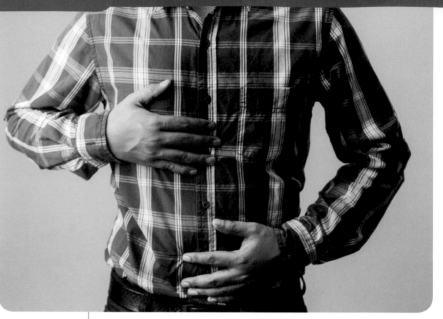

HEARTBURN

Boy, oh boy, did you do it this time. You added that heaping second helping to all the platter pickings you couldn't resist, and what do you have? Indigestion (an incomplete or imperfect digestion), that's what. And it may be accompanied by pain, nausea, vomiting, heartburn, gas, and belching. All this because you couldn't resist temptation. But don't worry. It happens to everybody, and it goes away.

So, now that you've eaten until you're about ready to burst, what's next? The couch, maybe? Stretch out, let your digestive system do its thing, take a nap?

Wrong! The worst thing you can do after a binge is to lie down. That can cause heartburn, also known as acid indiges-

tion. Whatever you call it, it's the feeling you get when digestive acid escapes your stomach and irritates the esophagus, the tube that leads from your throat to your stomach. After you eat, heartburn can also fire up when you:

- Bend forward
- Exercise
- Strain muscles

Why Acid Backs Up

Occasionally the acid keeps on coming until you have a mouthful of something bitter and acidy. You may have some pain in your gut, too, or in your chest.

Along with that acid may come a belch, one that may bring even more of that stomach acid with it.

The purpose of stomach acid is to break down the foods we eat so our body can digest them. Our stomachs have a protective lining that shields it from those acids, but the esophagus does not have that protection. Normally that's not a problem, because after we swallow food, it passes down the esophagus, through a sphincter, and into the stomach. The sphincter then closes.

WHEN TO CALL THE DOCTOR

Food poisoning can be debilitating for a day or two, but you'll start feeling better after the poison leaves your system. Sometimes, though, food poisoning can be very dangerous. If you have any of these symptoms, see a doctor immediately:

- Diarrhea and vomiting that last more than 48 hours
- A fever over 101°F
- Stomach cramps that keep getting worse
- Blood in your stool
- Dehydration
- Stiff neck, severe headache, and fever

An important note: If the person poisoned is a young child, an elderly person, or someone with an impaired immune system (they're just getting over an illness or they have a more serious condition such as AIDS), see the doctor at the first sign of food poisoning.

Occasionally, though, the muscles of that sphincter are weakened and it doesn't close properly or it doesn't close all the way. Scarring from an ulcer or frequent episodes of acid reflux (when the acid comes back up), stomach pressure from overeating, obesity, and pregnancy can all cause this glitch in the lower esophageal sphincter (LES). And when the LES gets a glitch and allows the gastric acid to splash out of the stomach, you get heartburn.

Generally, heartburn isn't serious. In fact, small amounts of reflux are normal and most people don't even notice it because the swallowing we do causes saliva to wash the acids right back down into the stomach where they belong. When the stomach starts shooting back amounts that are larger than normal, especially on a regular basis or over a prolonged period of time, that's when the real trouble begins, and simple heartburn can turn into esophageal inflammation or bleeding.

Who's prone to heartburn? Just about anybody. According to the National Digestive Diseases Clearinghouse, 25 million adults suffer from heartburn daily and about 60 million Americans get gastroesophageal reflux and heartburn at least once a month.

There are several prescription medicines available for the treatment of long-term or serious heartburn or acid reflux, and over-the-counter remedies are available at your pharmacy, too. But there are several remedies right in your own kitchen that can fight the fire of heartburn.

From the Cupboard

Almonds. Chewing 6 or 8 blanched almonds during an episode of heartburn may relieve the symptoms. Chew them well, though, to avoid swallowing air and causing yourself more discomfort.

GUM CHEWERS

Gum-chewers are notorious air-swallowers. And air-swallowers are prone to indigestion. So if you're a gum-chewer who gets frequent indigestion, skip the gum for awhile to see if there's a connection.

If you already are suffering with a bout of heartburn, however, chewing sugarless gum can bring relief. It increases the flow of saliva, which washes down the acid. Skip the mint flavors and don't chew too much because that can lead to air-swallowing.

Baking soda. Take ½ teaspoon in ½ glass water. Check the antacid use information on the box before using this remedy, however. Warning! If you're on a salt-restricted diet, do not use baking soda. It's loaded with sodium. And do not use it if you're experiencing nausea, stomachache, gas, cramps, or stomach distention caused by overeating.

Brown rice. Plain or with a little sweetening, rice can help relieve discomfort. Rice is a complex carbohydrate and is a bland food, which is less likely to increase acidity or relax the sphincter muscle.

Cream of Tartar. For an acid neutralizer, mix ½ teaspoon with ½ teaspoon baking soda in a glass of water. Take 1 teaspoon of the solution as needed.

Soda crackers. This is an old folk cure that actually works. Soda crackers (preferably unsalted) are bland, they digest easily, and they absorb stomach acid. They also contain bicarbonate of soda and cream of tartar, which neutralize the acid.

> ## FASCINATING FACT
>
> Cold beverages may help cause heartburn. They cool down your stomach, which requires a certain amount of heat in order to function at its best.

Tip: You know that package of soda crackers they always give you at the restaurant, that you leave on the table? From now on, take them with you. These come in handy when you're plagued by heartburn and can't seek immediate relief.

Vinegar. Mix 1 tablespoon apple cider vinegar, 1 tablespoon honey, and 1 cup warm water. Drink at the first sign of heartburn.

From the Drawer

Paper and pen. Keep a food diary. This can tell you which foods or food combinations cause that heartburn.

From the Faucet

Water. Drink water in between meals, not with meals. If you drink fluids with meals, you increase the volume of stomach contents, which makes it easier for heartburn to happen.

From the Refrigerator

Apples. They cool the burn of stomach acid. Eat them fresh, with the skin still on, or cook them for desserts.

Apple honey. This is a simple remedy that will neutralize stomach acids. Peel, core, and slice several sweet apples. Simmer with a little water over low heat for three hours until the mixture is thick, brown, and sweet to the taste. Refrigerate in an airtight container and take a few spoonfuls whenever you have the need.

Buttermilk. This is an acid-reliever, but don't confuse it with regular milk, which can be an acid-maker, especially if you are bothered by lactose intolerance.

Cabbage. Like apples, this is a natural fire extinguisher for stomach burn. For the best relief, put the cabbage through a juicer, then drink it.

Fruit juices. Skip juices from citrus fruits, but try these stomach-cooling juices for heartburn relief: papaya, mango, guava, pear.

Lime juice. Mix 10 drops lime juice with $\frac{1}{2}$ teaspoon sugar and $\frac{1}{4}$ teaspoon baking soda, in that order. When the baking soda is added it will fizz, and that's when you need to drink it down. The fizz will neutralize stomach acid.

Papaya. Eat it straight to reap the benefit of its natural, indigestion-fighting enzyme papain. Or drink 1 cup papaya juice combined with 1 teaspoon sugar and 2 pinches cardamom to relieve acid. Warning! Pregnant women should not eat papayas; they're a source of natural estrogen that can cause miscarriage.

Potato. Mix $\frac{1}{2}$ cup raw potato juice with $\frac{1}{2}$ cup water, and drink after meals. To make raw potato juice, simply put a peeled raw potato through a juicer or blender.

Pumpkin. Eat it baked as a squash to get rid of heartburn. Fresh is best. Spice it up with cinnamon, which is another heartburn cure. Or, make a compote of baked pumpkin and apples, spiced with cinnamon and honey, for a dessert that's both curative and tasty.

Yogurt. Make sure it has live cultures in it. Because of the helpful and digestive-friendly microorganisms in yogurt, it may sooth the acid-forming imbalances that can lead to heartburn.

From the Spice Rack

Cardamom. This old-time digestive aid may help relieve the burn of acid indigestion. Add it to baked goodies such as sweet rolls or fruit cake, or sprinkle, with a pinch of cinnamon, on toast. It works well in cooked cereals, too.

Cinnamon. This is a traditional remedy for acid relief. Brew a cup of cinnamon tea from a cinnamon stick. Or try a commercial brand, but check the label. Cinnamon tea often has black tea in it, which is a cause of heartburn, so make sure your commercial brand doesn't contain black tea. For another acid-busting treat, make cinnamon toast.

Ginger. A tea from this root can soothe that burning belly. Add 1 $\frac{1}{2}$ teaspoons ginger root to 1 cup water; simmer for ten minutes. Drink as needed.

Sage. For a tea that can relieve stomach weakness that allows acid to be released back into the esophagus, take 2 $\frac{1}{2}$ cups boiling water, $\frac{1}{4}$ cup fresh sage leaves, 1 teaspoon sugar or honey, and the juice of $\frac{1}{2}$ lemon. Combine ingredients and steep for 20 minutes. Strain and drink while it's warm.

Fire-Fighting Foods

Proteins may strengthen the sphincter that allows the stomach acid to escape. Make sure all your meals contain some protein in order to keep that valve in good working order. These top the sphincter-friendly list:

- Lean meats
- Fish
- Poultry

- Low fat dairy products

More Do's and Don'ts

- If you're carrying extra pounds, lose them. All that baggage pushing in on the abdomen increases pressure on the stomach, which causes heartburn.

- Eat smaller meals. The more food in your belly, the more likely that bulk will push stomach acid right back up.

- Eat slowly, chew thoroughly. Sometimes heartburn will flare because the food is simply too large to get through the digestive tract and it, along with

WHEN TO CALL THE DOCTOR

- If you've tried home remedies or over-the-counter medications and they're not working. Your heartburn could be a symptom of another ailment, such as an ulcer, gallbladder disease, or hiatal hernia.

- If heartburn happens on a prolonged or regular basis, even if home treatments are working

- Call 9-1-1 or go to the nearest emergency room if you're experiencing chest pain that spreads into your arm, jaw, or shoulder, especially when accompanied by any of these symptoms: sweating, nausea, dizziness, shortness of breath, fainting. This could be a heart attack

the acids, is forced back up.

- Don't eat right before bedtime. Give your stomach a two- or three-hour break before you sleep. And if you're plagued by the burn at night, sleep with your head elevated on pillows.

- Let the gravity be with you. Stay upright so the gastric contents are forced to stay down. In other words, don't head for the couch after you eat. If you must snooze, try the recliner, but don't recline too steeply.

- Loosen the belt. Tight clothing and belts can create enough pressure to cause heartburn.

- Stay in shape. Heartburn hates people who are fit. However, skip strenuous exercise for a couple hours after a meal. Instead, go for a nice leisurely walk. This helps keep the stomach acid in its place.

- Stay calm. Stress increases acid production.

Herbal Remedies

Aloe vera gel. Mix 2 tablespoons aloe vera gel with a pinch of baking soda for quick heartburn relief.

Chicory. This herb is an acquired taste and is found most commonly in coffee. It can neutralize acid indigestion. Brew up a little tea with 3 tablespoons chicory root and 1 quart boiling water. Let it cool completely, then drink a cup whenever it becomes necessary.

The Usual Suspects

Here's the food list that's commonly associated with heartburn. Cut back on these, or cut them out altogether, and see what happens:

Fried and fatty foods, pies, cakes, cookies, butter, margarine, oils, cream: These may weaken your LES. Also, fatty foods take longer to digest, meaning the gastric juices are working overtime and have more opportunity to cause a backup.

Peppermint in any form: It relaxes the stomach muscle and valve, allowing the release of acids back up into the esophagus. Warning! Peppermint is often prescribed for other symptoms of indigestion but should never be used when heartburn is present as well.

Caffeinated beverages, such as coffee, tea, cola: Caffeine causes extra acid production.

Chocolate: It contains methylxanthines, a second cousin to caffeine, and can weaken the stomach valve.

Fruit and vegetable juices, especially tomato and citrus juice: They can irritate the throat and cause pain if heartburn has already caused irritation. Pineapple juice has an especially potent punch.

Garlic and onions: May weaken the LES.

Spicy, pickled, or fermented foods: These are heartburn-makers, too.

Alcohol: It causes the LES to relax.

Smoking and certain drugs such as aspirin, ibuprofen, and some antibiotics: These also relax the LES, causing acid reflux.

LARYNGITIS

Have you been verbally abusing your voice? Too much vocal enthusiasm at a sports event can set you up for swollen vocal cords and no voice the next day. But that's not the only way to cause laryngitis—the result of inflammation of the voice box and voice folds. More often, laryngitis is caused by an upper respiratory infection, usually viral, such as the common cold. Surprisingly, some cases of laryngitis are caused by heartburn, especially in the elderly. During the night, the acid-rich contents of the stomach come back up the throat and then cause irritation.

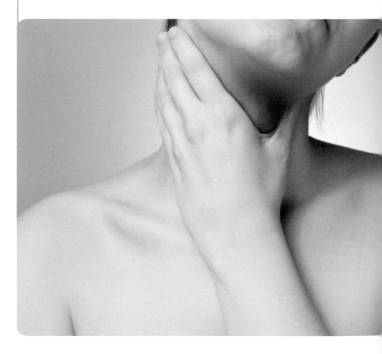

Sounds and Symptoms

When we speak, two membranes, known as the vocal chords, vibrate to produce sounds. Hoarseness, the main sign of laryngitis, is an indicator that something with the vocal chords is wrong, swollen, irritated, or infected. Besides hoarseness, symptoms of acute, or short-term, laryngitis also include a painful or scratchy feeling in the throat, a loss of range in the voice, and fatigue. You may also have the annoying feeling that you must constantly clear your throat. In heartburn-induced laryngitis, symptoms include waking up with a bad taste in the mouth, feeling like something is sticking in the throat, constant throat clearing, and hoarseness that gradually improves during the day.

From the Cupboard

Salt. A saltwater gargle helps heal infected and inflamed vocal chords and sore throats. Add ½ teaspoon salt to 1 cup warm water and gargle several times a day as needed. Be careful to use the correct amount of salt. Gargling with a solution as salty as the sea will only increase the irritation.

LOOK LIKE AN ELEPHANT, TALK LIKE A HORSE

Here's a way to transform yourself into an elephant man or woman: Drink lots of alcohol. Excessive drinking over a period of time causes chronic laryngitis and some unsightly elephantlike features. No, you won't sprout Dumbo ears, but the folds of your vocal cords will resemble elephant skin, hence the medical name pachydermia from the term pachyderm, meaning thick skinned. Wrinkled and tough vocal cords result in a voice that is gravelly, hoarse, and often unintelligible.

Vinegar. Viruses and bacteria dread an acidic environment, so why not make your mouth one big, albeit weak, acid bath? Gargling with vinegar, a weak acid, can help wipe out many infectious organisms. Pour equal amounts of vinegar and water into a cup, mix, and gargle two to four times a day. You can also gargle with straight vinegar, but some people find it too strong, especially at first.

From the Refrigerator

Lemon. Some folk remedies require you to suck on a lemon to cure a sore throat. An impossible task, indeed! Spare yourself the face-contorting agony and try a lemon juice and salt gargle instead. Lemon is naturally acidic and helps stimulate saliva flow. The salt increases the lemon's acidity, which in turn helps kill many microorganisms prone to weak acids. To make this gargle, juice a whole lemon into a bowl and add a pinch of sea salt (or regular salt). Mix well. Add 1 teaspoon of the concentrated lemon-salt mixture to 1 cup warm water. Gargle three to four times a day as needed.

From the Sink

Soap and water. Laryngitis can be caused by a viral infection and is easily spread by hand-to-hand contact or by touching contaminated surfaces. Avoiding such germs is one of the best ways to prevent laryngitis. If you or someone around you has a cold, be extra vigilant about washing your hands with warm water and soap. Clean common surfaces, such as the telephone and door handles, with vinegar and a clean cloth.

Water. Keep the throat moistened and stay hydrated by drinking your daily amount of water (eight, 8-ounce glasses per day). Fruit juices also fit the bill, as do hot, noncaffeinated drinks, which may feel extra soothing on sore throat tissues.

From the Spice Rack

Garlic. Should you have a strong stomach and no social events to attend, try what the Amish and Seventh Day Adventists suggest for treating sore

WITCH HAZEL TO THE RESCUE

The bark, leaves, and twigs of witch hazel are high in tannins, giving this plant astringent properties. Astringents are substances that can dry, tighten, and harden tissues...perfect for shrinking swollen throat tissues. A throat gargle of store-bought witch hazel, myrrh, and cloves helps reduce the pain of sore throats associated with laryngitis. Place 1 dropper full of tincture of each herb in a sip of water and rinse. If myrrh and cloves aren't available, dilute witch hazel with 3 parts water and rinse. Do not swallow the mixture.

throats and viral infections: Suck on a slice of garlic. Garlic, when sliced or crushed, releases the antimicrobial substance allicin. Allicin kills bacteria, including strep and some viruses. Slice a garlic clove down the middle and place half a clove on each side of the mouth. Pretend the cloves are lozenges and suck on them. Use as often as necessary, or as often as you can handle garlic breath.

Ginger. Fragrant, fresh ginger can help soothe inflamed mucous membranes of the larynx. Try sucking on candied ginger if available or drink a cup of ginger tea. To prepare the tea, cut a fresh 1– to 2 – inch gingerroot into thin slices and place in 1 quart boiling water. Cover the pot and simmer on the lowest heat for 30 minutes. Let cool for 30 more minutes, strain, and drink $\frac{1}{2}$ to 1 cup three to five times a day. Sweeten with honey if needed.

WHEN TO CALL THE DOCTOR

- If pain is present with hoarseness
- If the hoarseness continues for more than 72 hours
- If you have an upper-respiratory infection with fever that lasts more than a couple of days
- If you have trouble breathing
- If you notice a permanent change in the pitch of your voice, especially if you are a smoker
- If you cough up blood

From the Stove

Steam. Dry indoor air, so common in the wintertime, combined with an irritated throat can make you extra miserable. Start the day off steamy. Bring half a pot of water to boil, remove from stove, and place on a protected surface. Drape a towel over your head, lean forward over the pot, and breathe gently for 10 to 15 minutes. Be careful not to stick your face too close. Repeat in the evening before bedtime.

More Do's and Don'ts

- Don't smoke, and stay out of smoky environments. Smoking and breathing secondhand smoke irritate the larynx and cause coughing, which only adds more pain to the picture. Smoking, by the way, is one of the most common causes of chronic laryngitis.

- Avoid alcohol, since it dehydrates the body and can cause long-term vocal problems if abused.

- Cut back on coffee. Same goes for caffeinated teas and soft drinks. Caffeine, like alcohol, sucks out moisture from the body, so it's a big no-no if you suffer from heartburn-induced laryngitis. Caffeine actually relaxes the muscles and valves that control the stomach's entrance (the lower esophageal sphincter).

- Avoid whispering, as it can further irritate the throat. Soothe your vocal chords by speaking in a soft, modulated voice. Better yet, don't even try to talk. Communicate via the written word when possible.

- Don't constantly clear your throat. This only bothers the vocal chords—and the person next to you. If your throat feels like it needs clearing, try gargling with warm water or with salt water instead.

- At night, run a humidifier in your room. Remember to clean it frequently.

- Be kind to your voice. Bring a noise-maker to pep rallies and use it instead of screaming. Buy a whistle to call your kids in from play. Cheer the team using hand and body signals or big cardboard signs.

- Save dusting for another day. Dust particles aren't friendly to a sore throat.

- When in an ultra-dry environment, such as an airplane, make sure you stay extra hydrated. Drink more than the normal amount of water, and snack on waterlogged fruits or vegetables, such as grapes, melons, or celery sticks.

STOMACH UPSET

You and the wife celebrated your promotion with dinner at your favorite bar becue joint. You've been working hard for months, you think, so you deserve to cut loose a little. On the way home you groan and mutter that you wish you had stopped after that first barbecue platter. Your wife shrugs her shoulders. You both know the price for your revelry will be a subsequent painful night of bloating, gas, and heartburn.

But sometimes your tummy can turn on you even when you haven't been making one too many trips to the buffet table. It's important to know what's normal tummy trouble and what's something to take more seriously.

The Digestive Dance

When you eat something, the digestive process begins right away in your mouth. Your salivary glands produce digestive juices that lubricate your food and prepare fat for digestion. The food travels through your esophagus into your stomach, where digestive juices continue to break food down even further so it can travel on to the small intestine. The pancreas and liver secrete other digestive juices that flow into the small intestines. In the small intestine, vital nutrients including vitamins, minerals, water, salt,

STOMACH? YOU ARE HERE

You're on a game show and the host asks the million dollar question. Where is your stomach located? If you're like most people, you'd say in the center of your abdomen. Unfortunately, you'd be out a lot of money if you made that your final answer. The stomach is actually much higher than you think. It's located under the ribs just to the left of your sternum.

carbohydrates, and proteins are sucked out of the food and absorbed into your body. By the time your dinner makes its way to the large intestines, it's mostly bulk and water. The large intestines absorb the water and help you get rid of the, umm, excess.

But sometimes things in the digestive system go awry and cause indigestion, a catchall term that means you simply have trouble digesting your food. When you eat too much, or you eat the wrong foods, you may get one of a number of indigestion symptoms mentioned above: nausea, vomiting, heartburn, bloating, or gas. Those unpleasant feelings may send you running to the drugstore for relief, and if they do, you've got plenty of company. The American Gastroenterological Association says that digestive problems are one of the most common reasons Americans take over-the-counter medications. Indigestion can be a symptom of something more serious, such as gastritis, an ulcer, severe heartburn, irritable bowel syndrome, or diverticulitis. But if it's just the result of overdoing it at dinner, try some of these kitchen cures for a bit of relief.

From the Cupboard

Baking soda. Make your own antacid with baking soda. Mix $\frac{1}{2}$ teaspoon baking soda in $\frac{1}{2}$ glass water and drink away. But remember to read the antacid instructions on the baking soda label before you take this home remedy.

Crackers. You haven't eaten anything all day, and you can't understand why your stomach is churning and burning. The answer is probably overactive stomach acids. And your best bet is to eat something but to stick with something bland, such as nibbling on crackers.

Rice. If an overflow of stomach acid bothers you, try eating $\frac{1}{2}$ cup cooked rice with your dinner. It's a complex carbohydrate that keeps the stomach busy churning, diverting excess acid. Plus it's a bland food that tends to be easy on the stomach.

From the Drawer

Antacid. Antacids can help neutralize stomach acids, which can cut that burning sensation you feel when you have an empty stomach. But be careful what kind of antacid you choose. Though they help keep those stomach acids calm, antacids can cause other trouble if you're not careful. Most antacids have calcium or magnesium as a main ingredient. If you tend to be constipated, try an antacid with magnesium listed first on the list of ingredients. If diarrhea tends to be more bothersome for you, pick an antacid with calcium listed first.

From the Fruit Basket

Banana. If you have a sensitive tummy, bland foods such as bananas seem to ease the pain. One study found that half the people who took banana powder capsules every day for two months eased their tummy pain. You can get similar results by eating a banana—or better yet a plantain banana—every day.

LIFE AND TIMES OF YOUR LUNCH

You ate tuna fish on rye at noon, and that tuna will be with you for a while before it's digested. Take a look at how long food takes to get from entrance to exit.

Esophagus: One bite slides down the esophagus in eight seconds.

Stomach: Carbohydrates take two hours to digest. Proteins take four hours. Fatty foods stick around for six hours.

Small Intestines: Foods stay in this winding road for three to five hours.

Large Intestines: That sandwich will stay in the staging room of the large intestines for 4 to 72 hours before it makes its departure.

From the Refrigerator

Apple. Adding fiber to your diet will help alleviate stomachaches and keep your digestive system healthy. One study of fiber's effect on the tummy discovered that people who ate fiber-rich foods at the first sign of a tummyache cut their chances of getting a full-blown upset stomach in half. If you haven't been eating much fiber, be sure to start slowly. Jumping in with loads of fiber-rich foods after living on burgers and fries will give you a mean case of gas. Add fiber gradually over a few months and drink plenty of water to avoid overloading your system. To get started, grab an apple and nosh away, but remember to eat the peel—that's where you get most of your roughage.

Soda pop. Sipping on a can of de-caffeinated soda can help settle your stomach. This trick is especially useful if you've eaten too much. The carbonation in the soda causes you to burp, which is the quickest way to get relief from an overfull belly.

Water. Drinking water is your best bet for avoiding tummy trouble. It helps move things through the digestive system smoothly. Try drinking at least six to eight 8-ounce glasses of water a day.

From the Spice Rack

Caraway seeds. These seeds act very similarly to fennel seeds. They help with digestion and gas. You can either make a tea from the seed or you can do what people in Middle Eastern countries have done for centuries—simply chew on the seeds after dinner. Caraway seed tea: Place 1 teaspoon caraway seeds in a cup and add boiling water. Cover the cup and let stand for ten minutes. Strain well and drink up to 3 cups a day—be sure to drink on an empty stomach.

Cinnamon. This aromatic spice stimulates the digestive system, helping things move along the digestive tract smoothly. You can make a cinnamon tea by stirring $\frac{1}{4}$ to $\frac{1}{2}$ teaspoon cinnamon powder into 1 cup hot water. Let the tea stand for up to five minutes and drink.

Fennel seeds. This remedy is one of the most prescribed for gas and stomach cramps by medical herbalists. Try a fennel tea for your stomach: Place 1 teaspoon fennel seeds in a cup and add boiling water. Cover the cup and let stand for ten minutes. Strain well and drink up to 3 cups a day—be sure to drink on an empty stomach.

Ginger. Ginger is a long-time helper for stomach ailments of all types—particularly nausea and gas. Ginger helps food flow smoothly through the digestive tract, allowing the body to better absorb nutrients. Drink a cup of ginger tea to get your stomach back on track. To make your own ginger tea: Add $\frac{1}{2}$ teaspoon ground ginger to a cup of hot water, let stand for up to three minutes, strain, and drink away.

Mint. A folk remedy for indigestion, mint (in the form of peppermint or spearmint) can soothe a troubled tummy. Mint helps food move through the intestines properly and eases stomach cramps. Sip a cup of mint tea to let the herb work its magic: Put 1 teaspoon dried mint in a cup and add boiling water. Cover the cup and let it stand for ten minutes. Strain and drink up to 3 cups of the warm tea a day. Be sure to drink it on an empty stomach, and do not use this as a remedy if you have accompanying heartburn.

Thyme. Thyme stimulates the digestive tract, helps with stomach cramping, and relieves gas pressure. Try some thyme in a bottle (or cup) for your tummy trouble: Place 1 teaspoon dried thyme leaves in a cup. Fill the cup with boiling water and let stand, covered, for ten minutes. Strain and drink on an empty stomach up to three times a day.

IS BITTER BETTER?

Folk medicine has a grocery list of herbs that can ease stomach trouble and help your digestive system work like a dream, or at least a lot better than it has been. One of the most frequently recommended categories of digestive aids is a bitter tonic. These tonics help stimulate the digestive system by kicking in stomach acid and liver bile, which improve digestion and help the body better absorb essential nutrients. Some of the most frequently prescribed bitter tonic herbs are wormwood, chamomile, goldenseal, Oregon grape root, gentian, and boneset. Take note: Don't try a bitter tonic if you have heartburn or any other kind of pain with digestion.

From the Stove

Hot water. Heat some water on the stove and pour it into a hot water bottle. Put the soothing heat on your stomach after you eat to help increase circulation to the abdominal area. The improved circulation should help improve digestion.

More Do's and Don'ts

German researchers wanted to know what foods caused the most trouble for people. So they asked people what foods tended to create an aching tummy. The top three offenders for normal, healthy eaters were mayonnaise, cabbage, and fried and salted foods.

Avoid milk. Though many people think milk can soothe an aching tummy, it actually may do more harm than good. People who are lactose intolerant have trouble digesting milk and end up with bloating, gas, and cramping.

Cut the coffee. Coffee causes stomach irritation in some people.

Ax the alcohol. Alcohol is also a stomach irritant. If you have a sensitive tummy, skip the after-dinner drink.

Pass on pepper. Red or black pepper may add a kick to food, but it can also kick you in the tummy. Avoid it if it bothers your stomach.

Choose produce carefully. Some vegetables and fruits are notorious for their ability to produce tummy trouble. Watch out for broccoli, cabbage, brussels sprouts, and melons.

Wash your beans. Beans are the "musical fruit," but you can take the music out of them. Let them soak overnight in water, then drain the water and replace it with fresh water before cooking. Rinse canned beans, too. This simple technique will help avert gassy problems.

Get busy. Exercise helps get your digestive system moving as it should.

Banish the aspirin. Aspirin and nonsteroidal anti-inflammatory drugs such as ibuprofen have been known to cause ulcers. If you're prone to tummy trouble, avoid both of these drugs.

Relax. Many people get stomach troubles because they react poorly to stress. Don't let your worries add up to health issues for you. Learn some techniques for relaxing your mind and body.

Eat up. Don't skip meals. It allows acid to build up in your stomach and can leave you with an aching tummy.

Quit smoking. Smoking makes you more at risk for painful heartburn.

Slow down. Take time to enjoy your meal and allow your food to digest properly.

Herbal Remedies

Here are a couple herbal remedies for digestive ills.

Catnip. Used to treat digestive

WHEN TO CALL THE DOCTOR

- If you have excessive abdominal cramping that doesn't go away after 30 minutes or gets worse with time. You may have an intestinal obstruction.
- If you have vomiting, fever, extreme nausea, or abdominal cramping. You could have food poisoning or an ulcer.
- If your stomachache lasts for longer than a day
- If your indigestion is accompanied by pressure in the chest, nausea or vomiting, sweating, or breathing trouble. You could be having a heart attack.

problems, stomach cramps, and gas for hundreds of years, catnip has long been known as an aid for tummy trouble.

Like chamomile, catnip has sedative properties that help you—and your stomach—relax. Sip a cup of catnip tea when you are experiencing stomach upset: Place 1 teaspoon dried catnip in a cup and pour boiling water over the herb. Let the tea steep for ten minutes. Strain and drink up to 3 cups a day on an empty stomach.

Chamomile. This herb is well-known for its soothing properties. And it indeed eases stomach cramps and gas, basically helping the stomach relax. To make your own chamomile tea: Put 1 tablespoon chamomile flowers in a cup. Pour boiling water over the flowers and let sit for ten minutes. Strain and drink the warm tea on an empty stomach up to three times a day.

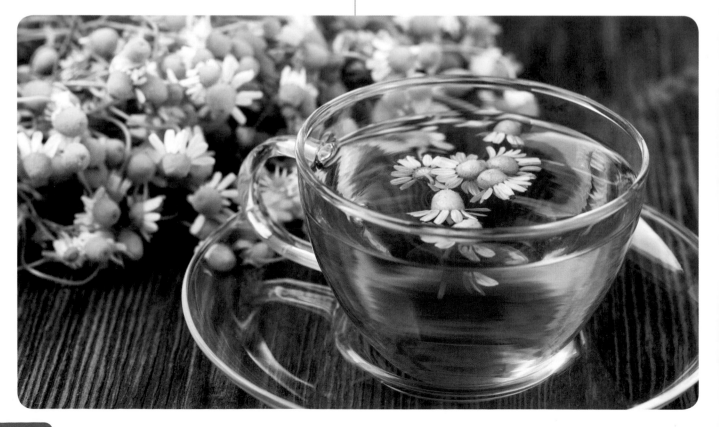